How To Stick To A Diet

Weight Loss Tips for Women

Emma J. Adams

ISBN-13: 978-0-9791653-5-1
ISBN-10: 0-9791653-5-0

First Printing, 2012

Printed in the United States of America

Creative Bookworm Press, Tucson AZ USA

Liability Disclaimer

The information provided here offers an educational resource only and is not intended to serve as nutritional, dietary, health, or medical advice related to any person's specific diet or health problems. There can be no assurance that any person's specific diet or health problems, diseases, or symptoms will heal, recover, or otherwise resolve as a result of applying the information provided here or in other resources mentioned in the book.

There also can be no assurance of safety with or absence of possible harm from any specific strategy, treatment or therapy if a specific person tries such treatment or therapy mentioned in this book, or other media. The reader is advised to seek personalized advice from a qualified nutritionist, dietician, and/or health care provider before attempting to implement information provided in this book.

Neither the author nor the publisher assumes any responsibility for any errors or omissions. The author and publisher also specifically disclaim any responsibility or liability resulting from the use of any of the information discussed in this book.

Terms of Use

This is copyrighted material. Your purchase of this book gives you a non-transferable, "personal use" license. You do not have any resale rights or private label rights from this book purchase.

How To Stick To A Diet

Weight Loss Tips for Women

Table of Contents

List of Images

Photos listed below are used with a specific license from Photos.com

COVER IMAGE SUPPLIED BY JUPITERIMAGES

The Best Diet for Women

"Energy and persistence conquer all things."

-- Benjamin Franklin

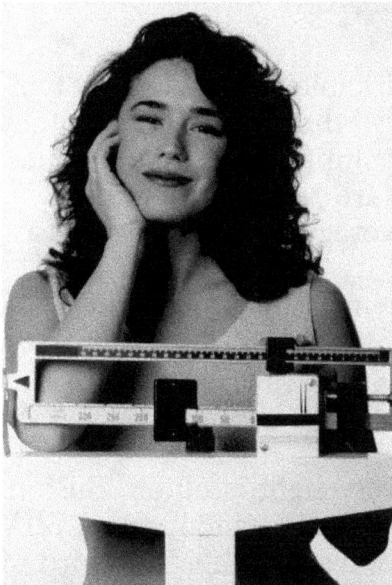

Sticking to a diet begins with planning and choosing the best diet for you.

What is the best diet for women?

The simplest answer is one that even the even the experts have finally discovered – the best diet is the one that you can stick with over the long haul.

That is, the best diet is a healthy diet for you, manageable – and appealing enough for you to stay on it most of the time.

Do you have to be perfect and never fall off the wagon?
No, you don't.

How "good "do you need to be?

If you are trying to lose some pounds fast, it turns out that you can lose more weight by eating a low carb menu (protein and good-for-you fats, veggies, and nuts) on only 2 days a week than if you struggle mightily to keep down your calories near starvation level every day of the week.

Yes. The diet that works is the one that you can stick with. This is real life, here, reality – not a reality show.

Of course, there is a lot more to it than just this simple point, but know that it is OK to be human. You can still lose weight.

Really.

Let's take a look at some remarkable facts – on any typical day in the U.S., almost half of the women say that they are on a diet. Women often compare themselves (unfavorably) with top models, who are 7 inches taller and over 20 pounds skinnier than the average woman in America.

Given the ideal put forth in the media, many women and girls see themselves as overweight or fat. Up to 10 million women suffer from some type of eating disorder in this country alone.

This isn't to say that being overweight is all an illusion. The National Center for Health Statistics found that 60% of adult women in the U.S. are overweight. One third of those overweight women are actually considered obese.

As a society, we are too sedentary, and we don't eat healthy nutritional diets overall. Foods that have too much sugar and salt, ridiculous quantities of fast food, and the use of junk food for comfort under stress all contribute to the problem. With age, overeating the empty calorie foods, and lack of regular exercise, we gain weight.

This book is for you to get the tips, tools, and tricks you need to succeed with the best diet for you. We will talk about how to choose the right diet, how to get proper support and encouragement, how to stay in control of cravings, and how to get back on track when you get lost for a while.

Let's get started...

You have probably asked this question of yourself many times, and you've probably also heard many other people say the same thing; why can't I seem to lose weight? (or the next question – even if I lose weight, why do I always end up putting it back on again?)

The simple fact that you're reading this information shows that you are still looking for a way to find the optimum body weight.

After trying many different diets and weight loss programs you might begin to think that you're a failure where the reality of the situation is that those very same diet and weight loss programs that you have tried have been the failures -- for you. They were not the right match for you and your complete situation.

They have failed to give you the desired results, not because of a lack of effort on your behalf, but more likely because they weren't targeting the cause of the problem.

Many diets and weight loss programs leave people feeling hungry for considerable times throughout the day. The hungrier you get, the more you want to eat. It becomes a survival thing.

Just as animals in the wild feel the need to eat when they are hungry, humans react in the same way. It is only natural that you should seek out food if you're feeling hungry. But − if you have not prepared for this inevitable hunt for food when you are hungry, you will end up grabbing whatever will fill you up, nutritious or not.

If your diet is supplying you properly with the right nutrients to meet your unique metabolism and energy needs, then you won't feel hungry all the time. Any weight-loss program that keeps you in such a state of hunger is destined to fail eventually, no matter how much willpower you might have.

It is simply not the natural state of human life.

That is one of the most common reasons why people can't seem to lose weight. Severe calorie restriction is just too hard to maintain, and it is detrimental to your health. You will eat up muscle instead of fat, get weak, and feel fuzzy headed. Your body will fight against the starvation message that it is getting.

Anybody can lose weight whether they have good willpower or not provided the body is getting sufficient nutritional requirements to eliminate hunger and to satisfy healthy functioning of the body...along with some other key tips that we will discuss later in this book.

Often women become overweight because they use food as a way to relax, celebrate, socialize, deal with sadness, enjoy happiness, and get through stressful situations.

But food is really innocent in all of this. It's just there to give you the energy you need to get through life. We add in all the meaning and power to a particular food.

And while food should taste good and be enjoyable, it shouldn't be the answer to all of your mental and emotional dilemmas. Instead, you need to find other outlets for dealing with your emotions.

There are several things you can do instead of finding comfort in food. For example:

- Take a hot bath

- Take a nap or just go to bed for the night

- Read

- Write in your journal

- Knit or crochet

- Listen to your favorite music

- Learn a new hobby

- Call a friend

- Play with your dog or cat

- Get a massage

- Drink a glass of water

- Have a good cry

- Hit a punching bag

- Take a walk

- Meditate

- Count to 10 – or 100 if necessary

When you learn some new activities to replace your dependence on food, you may find that you lose weight without even trying. You can still enjoy the food you eat, but you won't be dependent on it for your every need.

It's also important to break the habit of taking huge quantities of food at a meal and cleaning your plate. One trick that some authorities on dieting suggest is deliberately leaving at least the last forkful on your plate and pushing back from the table. Yes, you don't want to waste food in the big picture, but you don't really have to -- in the long run.

In the short run, if you want to change your usual eating habits, you need to do things just a little bit differently at first. Then, once you have established a new set of eating habits, you will find yourself eating smaller portions and being OK about finishing the portions you chose.

Easy Weight Loss Tips for Getting To Your Goals

If you've tried to lose weight and failed, you're probably thinking that it's a ridiculously difficult task to accomplish. You need some positive reinforcement here, something that tells you that you are on the right track.

Don't give up! Achieving your weight loss goals might be easier than you think!

Small Changes = Big Results

As you've no doubt realized, weight loss isn't a quick fix. You can't go on a two-week diet, lose the weight, and then think that the weight will stay off for good. Even if you're really good about following a diet at first, you'll more than likely gain the weight back.

Why?

It's because a two-week diet does nothing to alter your lifestyle, habits, mindset, or much else. It is as if you held your breath for 2 weeks and finally got to exhale and then breathe "normally."

But your "normal" eating patterns are not actually normal in the sense of being good for you, if they really contribute to keeping you above your ideal weight. They are just habits – and there are many ways to change habits.

Here's some good news - The best results come from changes that you incorporate into your daily life, and many of these changes aren't drastically different from what you do now.

You can even continue to enjoy many of the foods you love as long as you do so with a wise plan!

If you make a series of small changes, one at a time, you'll give yourself a chance to get used to them. It won't seem like such a shock to your system when you introduce the changes gradually.

Sooner than you think, you'll lose the weight and gain the healthy body and lifestyle that you desire!

And, if changing habits sounds a lot easier than it is for you, consider finding a good certified hypnotist or hypnotherapist in your area. Hypnosis is an excellent way to reprogram your mind to change habits in a lasting way.

Here are some weight loss tips to implement into your new lifestyle:

1. **Use low fat milk**. When you use low fat milk, you'll still get the nutritious benefits of milk, but without all the fat grams. Try substituting skim, 1%, or soy or unsweetened almond milk in your cereal, coffee, and cooking.

2. **Cut out soda**. Soda is a big offender when it comes to empty calories. The best thing you can do for your body is to replace the soda you're drinking with water. Water is critical to your good health.

Drinking enough water daily helps you clear toxins from your system, keeps your blood from clotting too easily, and may even lower your risk of heart attacks. It also helps fill you up and has zero calories, no matter how much you drink!

* If you're having trouble kicking the soda habit, try alternating soda and water each time you go to get a drink.

This will gradually get you used to less soda and increase your water intake.

If these ideas just aren't for you, think about making a great-tasting herb tea like raspberry or orange that you chill and add stevia as sweetener. No calories – and sometimes some extra health benefits. Some of the fruit flavored herb teas, for instance, include multiple herbs such as hibiscus – and hibiscus tea has been shown to help lower blood pressure.

Then, instead of making your weight worse and drinking pounds of sugar that contribute to your risk of diabetes and other health problems – you drink an herb tea that tastes sweet from the stevia, but that helps promote better health. Good deal!

3. **Start walking**. If a regular exercise routine is difficult for you, strive to walk more often. Walking doesn't feel so much like true exercise, but it is and you'll be rewarded for it. Wearing a simple pedometer to record your daily steps will give you useful feedback and encourage you to do a little more each day.

* Park farther from the store so you have to walk a little distance.

* Take the stairs instead of the elevator.

* Go for an enjoyable walk with your neighbor. You can visit, catch up, and exercise all at the same time!

* Take your dog out for a walk instead of just letting him out the door into the backyard.

* Walk around outside on your work breaks instead of snacking or sitting around the office.

* If you are on the phone at home, walk around while you are talking – don't sit. Sitting is bad for your health, and cordless/wireless phones make it simple to move around while you are on the phone.

4. **Watch your portion sizes**. Portion sizes just keep getting larger and larger, at least in restaurants. Don't buy into that.

You may not even realize that you're consuming a portion that's much too large for you. Look up what a healthy portion size really is for the meal you've chosen. You might be surprised at the results!

* Start your meals with a full glass of water.

* Combat oversized portions by using smaller plates.

* Half your plate should be vegetables, a quarter should be protein, and the other quarter should be carbohydrates.

* Give yourself the correct amount of food and then refrain from seconds.

5. **Have desserts sparingly**. Save desserts for special occasions or times when you deserve a nice treat. Avoid eating them every day, or you'll be adding massive amounts of calories to your daily intake. Or, if you just can't give up your treats, find low calorie versions of them

with a natural sweetener like stevia instead of artificial sweeteners or sugar.

* It's a good idea to plan ahead for occasional desserts and only buy them for those certain meals. That way, they aren't there tempting you the rest of the time.

* Have plenty of healthy snacks available to curb hunger or cravings in between meals. We'll talk more about the kinds of foods to have on hand later on.

⟡

You can easily turn these tips into healthy habits by incorporating them into your lifestyle one at a time. Get used to one tip before you add another one. Most of them involve only small changes. However, these small changes will enable you to achieve your weight loss goals!

By now, you may be wondering why we haven't talked about which diet is best for you. That's because you want to set yourself up to succeed, regardless of the diet plan you choose.

Diet is only one part of the equation. You need to set up the framework of your life to support your healthier eating lifestyle. That will include regular activity – not just exercise, but also a habit of standing up from sitting more often during a day, getting into an exercise routine, finding non-drug ways to support you and your sense of well-being, whether it is yoga or hypnosis or acupuncture (or all of the above).

Finally, there is one more important missing piece in choosing a diet that can succeed for you. We'll talk about that in the next chapter. It can make or break your ability to lose weight on a diet, or just to frustrate you...again.

Your Action Steps:

1. Decide which of the tips in this chapter make sense to you for your situation.

2. Implement them.

Food Addiction:
A Hidden Cause of Diet Failures

"We gain the strength of the temptation we resist."

- Ralph Waldo Emerson

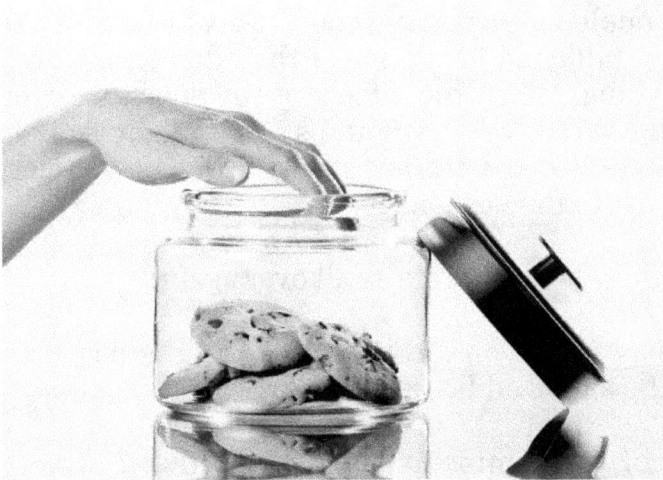

Food addiction is compulsive eating of foods that can cause some extreme ups and downs in your mood and physical symptoms. This also involves food cravings and, often, binges. Food binging can be as secretive as any alcoholic's or drug addict's binges.

Food addiction can also involve foods that you eat every day, as part of your regular diet. It does not just involve the obvious types of foods like sweets. You could be addicted to a long list of common foods and not know it.

Eating these foods may temporarily make you feel better. You might even get a short pick-me-up from eating a snack food that contains foods you are addicted to. Chocolate chip cookies, for instance, could include wheat, cane sugar or corn sugar, chocolate, egg, and milk.

If eating a food *seems* to relieve your afternoon fatigue or dullness or even makes a daily headache go away for a while, you may have found a trigger food. The ability of any food to change symptoms that you experience often is a warning sign of hidden food addiction.

The trouble is, every time you eat a source of the food(s) you are addicted to, you feed the addiction. You keep a cycle going. When the effects of the snack wear off, you develop withdrawal symptoms. You might feel sluggish and tired. You can't think straight. Maybe you get headaches. Until the next snack.

Then the whole cycle starts all over again.

You may not be an alcoholic or a drug addict – but you could be a food addict.

Some of the commonly-eaten foods that can be trigger foods for you are corn and corn sugar, wheat, yeast, milk, egg, beef, white potato, cane sugar, beet sugar, and chocolate. Many "junk foods" are addictive, but so are healthier versions of a particular food for a specific individual. For instance, the best organic whole wheat product can still be addictive, if the person is sensitized to wheat in any form.

It doesn't stop there. There are people who get addicted to all sorts of other foods, including some fruits or vegetables, various other types of animal proteins, beans, or soy.

The faster absorbed the food, the more likely it is to set this addictive cycle into motion. Believe it or not, some people may prefer beer because of the interaction of the alcohol with the food sources from which it is made, such as barley (which is a close relative to wheat), brewers yeast, and hops.

Someone else enjoys wine because of the interaction of the alcohol (which is absorbed super fast) with the food source like grapes (and sugar in grapes) and other fermented foods (like yeast).

You may have heard about "sugar addiction" or "chronic systemic "yeast" infections. Often, the problems are more complex for people who have those types of health issues. They probably have many additional food addictions/intolerances (the flip side of a food addiction is a food intolerance) that they don't even recognize.

Testing for Addictive Trigger Foods

Testing for trigger foods is the best (and cheapest) way to figure out if you have a food addiction problem. A trigger food test requires you to eliminate all sources of the item from your diet for 4-7 days. Then eat a test meal of only that single food (no extra condiments or other foods in the meal). The only beverage with a food test meal is plain water.

Keep a journal of what you eat, when you eat it, and what happens in the 1-24 hours after the test meal. If the test item is a trigger food, you will likely have unmasked your addiction and will experience the food intolerance side of the story.

In other words, the test meal will cause a set of symptoms you had commonly experienced in the past. You mood might flip around from irritability to depression for no apparent reason. A few hours later, you might get fatigued and headachy. Your heart may feel like it's racing. After that, you might find your nose running for a while.

By the next day, all of that amazing sequence of symptoms could be gone.

Some foods are a little slow to trigger you – so you might need to do two consecutive test meals of something like wheat cereal (you can make this from hot wheat cereal).

Overall, trigger food tests can give you awareness that how previously unsuspected foods have been playing a role in chronic health problems of all types.

What's in it for you? Eliminating trigger foods will help you feel energetic, alert, clear-headed, and less likely to experience chronic physical symptoms like indigestion, headaches, fatigue, depression, muscle and joint pains.

And, of course, it will help you stick to your weight loss diet and actually lose weight.

Big note of caution: If you happen to have serious medical conditions such as (but not limited to) asthma or epilepsy, do not attempt food tests without close medical supervision. It is very possible that a trigger food for you could trigger a bad asthma attack or epileptic seizure. So,

24

as every reader should, you especially need to discuss your options with your doctor before trying to test any foods.

Using the Results of Your Trigger Food Tests

Once you identify a food that can set off symptoms, put it on the list to eliminate from your diet completely for at least 3 months. You can re-test it after the 3 month avoidance period ends.

If you again experience a flare of symptoms after a food re-test, leave it out of your diet again for another 3 months.

Keep re-checking how you stand with the food every few months until it appears OK to put back into your diet *occasionally*. "Occasionally" means just that – no more often than once in 4 to 7 days.

The most important point about reintroducing a food to which you were addicted and/or intolerant is to make sure that you do not slip back into eating the food every day.

If you resume eating a trigger food daily, you'll slip back into the addictive cycle – craving the food, feeling better temporarily when you eat it, and then getting withdrawal symptoms when its effects wear off. The cycle will come on gradually – you might not even realize what is happening until you step back and acknowledge that you are addicted...again.

It's actually like a heroin or opiate addict in endless cycles of highs and withdrawals. After a while, the highs are harder to get from a hit of the drugs, and it takes more of the drug to get high.

As a food addict, you eventually run into the same inability to get the "pick-me-ups" that the food used to bring. Eventually, you spend most of your time with the food intolerance side of the problem – the unpleasant physical symptoms, fatigue, and negative moods.

Food addiction is not just a metaphor. It is a real biological effect. Scientists have already shown that they can get animals addicted to table sugar (sucrose) – and it cross-sensitizes the same brain chemistry that amphetamine or cocaine can affect. The sugar-addicted animals get withdrawal symptoms and crave sugar just as much as a drug addict craves their drug of choice.

Sugar is not the only food with direct links to the brain chemistry of addiction. Did you know that the normal digestion of foods like wheat and milk generates peptide hormones called exorphins? Exorphins from foods act like the drug morphine or the natural internal opiate-like peptides in the brain called endorphins.

You may have heard about runners' highs. Intense exercise can activate endorphins and make an athlete feel exhilarated from running. Some runners will even admit to feeling addicted to exercise, experiencing withdrawal symptoms when an injury or bad weather prevents them from getting their daily "hit" from exercise.

Just as a runner might get into an addictive cycle to activate their internal endorphins, a food addict might end up caught in their own addictive cycle -- caused by the exorphins from the digestion of wheat and milk as well as by the release of internal brain endorphins that eating sweet or fatty foods can naturally trigger.

What Food Addiction Means for You on a Diet

Although it is true that some people have genetic tendencies to be overweight, your genes are NOT your destiny. Unless you let them be. New research shows that environmental and diet factors turn genes on and off. In short, what you eat plays with your genes, turning sets of them on and off.

Choosing the right non-addictive foods for you is likely to tilt the balance in your favor – to flip the switches on your genes in a good way for health. This could be the missing step toward setting yourself up for successful weight loss.

So, what does this all mean for you as a woman wanting to diet successfully? It means at least two main things:

(1) You cannot hope to lose as much weight as you might otherwise if you keep addictive trigger foods and beverages in your diet. These foods can lead to inflammation, pain, and water weight gain.

(2) The tough time that you have in the first few days to a week of any new diet is not just from reducing calories – it's literally food withdrawal.

The initial dieting blues/misery could be severe withdrawal symptoms from your trigger foods. The good news is that if you go into the diet armed with knowledge about which foods you absolutely must avoid, you can make the transition to a healthier diet a lot easier.

In fact, you probably would want to identify your main trigger foods with food testing before you try a weight loss diet of any type.

Once you have found the problem foods and eliminated them (or replaced them with non-addictive alternatives – e.g., plain brown rice-based rice cakes if you have problems from wheat and yeast based breads), any weight loss diet is going to go much more smoothly.

Just from taking action on this food addiction factor alone, you can set yourself on course for successful weight loss.

Can't take the withdrawal symptoms from foods? Find yourself a good local acupuncturist. One place to begin your search is at www.AcuFinder.com. Acupuncture can help with many different types of addictions and related symptoms. Some studies show that acupuncture can even help alcoholics and drug addicts get through their withdrawal periods more easily.

It's also often the case that complete elimination of a specific food for a period of 3-6 months or so can lower your sensitization level and allow you to reintroduce the food on a limited basis without setting off the cravings.

But, as we discussed above, if you do the elimination period and a test meal 3 months later still sets off cravings and symptom cycling, eliminate the food for another few months before re-testing.

Your Action Steps:

1. Talk to your doctor or primary health care provider about whether or not it would be safe for you to try some trigger food tests at home.

2. Eliminate each food that you discover to be a trigger food for mood swings, physical symptoms, fatigue, or pain (joint pain, muscle pain).

Leave it out of your diet plan for 3 months before you retest it.

3. Replace a problem food with a rarely-eaten item that you have not been eating very often.

So, for instance, you might find that rice based pastas, breads, etc. are OK, even if wheat based foods are not. Try almond milk instead of cow's milk if milk is an issue for you.

Is beef a factor in your joint pain? Rotate in some wild game meats like venison or elk, fish and turkey instead.

4. Then choose the weight loss program that best matches your lifestyle, preferences, and goals.

Remember, what matters is that it is a program that you can stick with. And it should promote a healthy body and mind with a set of eating habits that are good for you.

5. Get even more detailed help with food addiction.

Visit www.OvercomeFoodAddiction.com for news, updates, and a complete membership program.

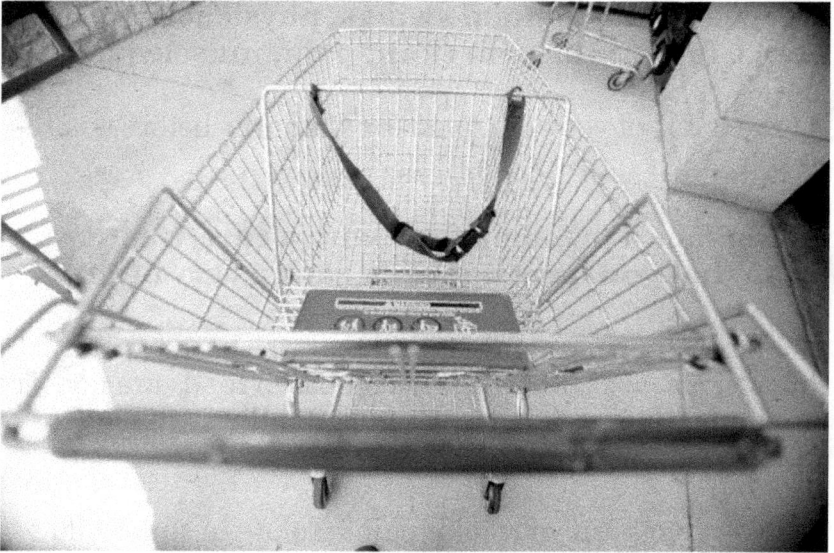

"With the new day comes new strength and new thoughts."

- Eleanor Roosevelt

Choosing Your Diet Plan

"Failing to plan is planning to fail." – Alan Lakein

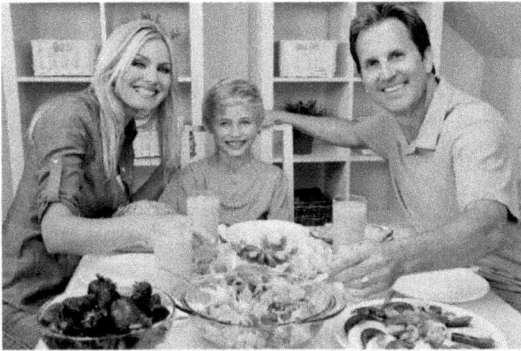

OK – now you are ready to choose the diet plan for you to lose weight and keep it off.

There are many different reasons that you might have decided to diet right now. You may be preparing for a big event. You may have made a big New Year's resolution. Or it may be that you're just ready to lose some weight to improve your health.

Most diets boil down to a set of strategies that give you fewer calories, eliminate junk foods, and restrict your intake of foods high in carbohydrates and/or fats. Every healthy diet includes eating lots of fresh vegetables that are the less starchy types.

31

The sources of the proteins that you choose are also important, since you only have 3 main macro-nutrients to fiddle around with in your diet: carbohydrates, fats, and proteins.

The evidence for their health promoting effects is really confusing. What we do know at this point is:

1. Lower carb diets are probably good choices for many people.

This type of diet reduces the intake of junk foods and items that can trigger you body to need to use the hormone insulin. If you don't release the insulin, your body does not have a chance to fail at using the insulin properly.

Inability to use insulin properly to get bodily cells to take up and use blood sugar correctly is the immediate reason why people develop diabetes. A frightening number of people in the U.S. and other developed countries have pre diabetes or diabetes type 2, with high blood sugar levels that damage organs throughout the body.

Resistance of the body's cells to the effects of insulin is the immediate cause of the high blood sugars that wreak havoc on your eyes, nerves, heart, blood vessels, kidneys, and more in these conditions. Being overweight contributes to the problem for a variety of reasons, but one factor is that fat seems to make it harder for insulin to do its job.

Are all carbs bad for you? Not at all. There is a lot to be said for low carb eating. Carbs in certain fruits like berries, for example, do not hit your blood sugar as hard as other fruits like bananas. And berries are full of antioxidants that can protect your cells from damage and promote health in other ways.

2. Low fat diets are less clearcut.

It is probably helpful to eliminate certain food sources of fats like red meats. But fatty fish like wild salmon has health-promoting omega-3 fatty acids.

This type of fat is good for you. Omega-3 fatty acids can improve your cholesterol, probably reduce your risks for heart attack and stroke, cut down inflammation all over the body, improve and stabilize mood, and more.

Experts argue, though, over saturated fats. Some people believe that all saturated fats are bad for you. Others point to studies suggesting that only some are. Monosaturated fats like olive oil, for instance, may be good for your heart health.

Fats are necessary to give you a feeling of satiety and stabilize your sense of hunger. If you feel full, it really helps cut down on your craving for foods and the risk that you will break down into a binge on forbidden foods.

3. High protein diets probably help you lose weight, but the scientific evidence is that balanced and complete vegetable proteins (e.g., beans complemented with a food source that has the amino acids that many beans may lack) are better for you than animal proteins as sources.

Remember to work with what you have learned about your own food addictions. Everyone is different, not only in what foods they like to eat, but also in which foods will help them lose weight.

Specific Foods To Help You Diet for Weight Loss and Health

When you think of losing weight, your first thought is naturally about the foods you will have to eliminate from your diet. But, how often do you think about the foods you need to add? Probably not very often.

While some diet and weight loss programs talk about eating less, others emphasize adding foods to your diet. Not just any foods, however. There are several foods considered to be very helpful for anyone trying to lose weight. Here are a few foods that are right at the top of the list.

Oatmeal

Oatmeal and oat bran are loaded with fiber and when eaten can expand to almost 30 times their volume. The combination of these two effects decreases your appetite by making you feel fuller longer. You can go for long periods of time without eating while keeping your energy levels high at the same time. In order to increase the effectiveness of your weight loss program, eat oatmeal about two hours before doing your workout.

Steel-cut oats, rolled oats, and plain or natural oatmeal are your best options. Avoid the instant flavored oatmeal in packets as they contain lots of sugar and other additives, and they are much more processed, meaning the fiber content is decreased.

Raw Fruits and Vegetables

Your body burns, on average, 15% more calories when your meals contain mostly raw fruits and veggies than if you ate a meal with no fruits or vegetables. It just makes sense, then, in order to lose weight you want to eat meals consisting of mostly raw ingredients.

Since these ingredients still have all of their nutrients, your body gets what it needs while you feel satisfied. Also, fruits and vegetables that are high in vitamin C, like lemons, oranges, berries, kiwis, and pineapple help your body to mobilize and flush out extra body fat.

Spices

For years, people have claimed that adding spices to your diet can help with weight loss. Recently, a professor at Oxford University found that by eating just 3 grams of chili peppers in a meal can increase your fat-burning metabolism by 8% to 20%, for up to three hours after eating the peppers.

Also, the addition of spicy mustard to your sandwich may burn an extra 45 to 75 calories over the same three hour time span. And, just by adding fresh ginger to your diet, you get a strong diuretic.

Fresh ginger also increases growth hormone production, therefore increasing the amount of fat released from your body's fat stores for burning as fuel.

Apples

While eating raw fruits in general is typically considered a great way to lose weight, apples are especially important to single out. Apples contain pectin, which prevents your body from over-absorbing fat, as well as causing your body to release some of the stored fat.

A study done in Brazil found that people who ate an apple before each meal lost 33% more weight than a group of people who didn't eat an apple. Pectin also acts as an appetite suppressant, so they are great snacks to tide you over between meals.

Fish

Not only are most fish loaded with tons of omega-3s, but fish like tuna, sardines, and salmon trigger the hormone leptin. Leptin is a fat-burning hormone that suppresses your appetite and determines whether you store the calories you eat as fat, or if you burn those calories for energy.

The origin of the word is interesting, too. Leptin originated from the Greek word "leptos" which means "slender." Adding more leptin to your diet may just prove to be slenderizing for you.

Eating certain foods to lose weight is not a brand new theory. We've often heard about diet fads that include one or two foods that dominate the program. The idea of eating specific foods that have been scientifically studied is a much more recent development in the weight loss world. When you look at the reasons why certain foods actually help you burn fat and calories, it just makes sense to add those foods to your diet plan.

Preparing for Success with your Diet

Whatever your reasons, starting a diet can be an exciting and invigorating idea. But after a few weeks, or even days, dieting isn't quite so appealing. You may be missing some of your old food choices, you may feel hungrier, or you may just feel deprived and angry.

But there are success strategies that will help you stick to your diet and reach your goals without stalling out. When you understand diet basics and tips for maintaining your progress, you'll reach your goal in no time.

Sticking to your diet actually starts with choosing your diet in the first place. There are thousands of diets you could try and it's important that you do your homework before you start one.

A diet needs to fit in with your lifestyle and be something that you can do realistically. For example, eating a diet of raw foods may be extremely healthy and help you lose weight. But it's not for everyone.

If you work two jobs it's probably not the best because of all the time-consuming food prep. If you don't have time to buy or prepare the appropriate foods, it's not likely that you'll stick to this diet for very long.

And there are hundreds more diets that have components that may not work for you while some diets will be perfect for you. So you must choose a diet that will not defeat you in the very beginning.

Here are a few things you should ask about a diet before beginning it:

• How much food preparation will be involved?

• Will you have to buy special products?

• Do you need specific tools that you don't already own?

• Is the food something you already like?

• Does this diet work with your current work schedule and lifestyle?

• Will you have to diet alone, or can your family also practice this way of eating?

• Will you be able to eat out? Or will all food have to come from home?

• How much money will you need spend each month for this diet?

• Will you have to attend meetings for it?

• Will the diet interfere with any health conditions or medications?

• Have you tried this diet before?

You want to choose a diet that fits within your budget and fits within your schedule. If you have a lot of free time, a diet that requires a lot of food preparation may be appropriate.

However, if you're very busy, you'll want to find a diet that you can fit into your erratic schedule. If you don't have time for a lot of food prep or you eat out a lot, you need to make sure your diet is compatible with these requirements.

This is an essential but practical step in sticking to your diet. If you choose a diet that fits well into your existing lifestyle, you'll have a better chance of continuing.

If you choose something that is difficult to fit into your lifestyle, you'll have more of a struggle ahead of you.

Choosing the Best Weight Loss Diet Plan for You

That four letter word 'diet' brings about all sorts of different emotions in people and more often than not those emotions tend to be negative. To most people a diet is a struggle.

It is something that they would rather not have to do. People only go on diets because they know that they have to do something about their weight and their health. It is a choice made out of necessity.

As soon as you believe you are on a diet you also become aware of the fact that you are going to get off it again and what do you expect will happen when you get off the diet that is helping you to get in shape?

For most people getting off a diet means reverting back to their former lifestyle and that is the lifestyle that got them overweight in the first place.

As we've already discussed, what you really should be doing is not dieting but making lifestyle changes because lifestyle changes are something that you can continue with forever.

If you make lifestyle changes that result in healthy body weight then you will maintain that body weight for as long as you maintain that lifestyle. It is not something that you will get off at the end of achieving a short-term result.

A lifestyle is a way that you intend to live for the long-term and that is how you will remain in good shape for the long-term.

$\diamond$

How often do you hear people saying that they are on a diet? And the next minute they are no longer on the diet. Stress or holidays or travel – whatever – come up and give them the excuse to quit the diet. Again.

What they should be saying is; I have made lifestyle changes and the result of those changes have been a reduction in body fat, an increase on my energy levels and an overall improvement in health.

That is what lifestyle changes can do for you and it is something that short-term diets rarely achieve.

Sleep and Weight Loss

Sleeping and eating are connected with one another. Really.

Many people don't realize that a lack of sleep can have a detrimental effect on your weight.

When you are constantly over tired your energy levels are naturally lacking and the first thing that most people do to boost their energy levels is to eat more food.

Eating more food is going to cause you to increase weight and the digestion of the food will burn up even more energy so you get into a vicious circle of tiredness, eating, and more tiredness.

The constant tiredness also affects the way that your body functions as it becomes less efficient and in doing so you tend to store more fat and gain weight.

Simply getting a bit more sleep at regular times at night can boost your energy levels and in doing so reduce your dependence upon food for energy and help you to lose weight without having to go on any diets.

If there are no alternatives to your lack of sleep due to circumstances in your life then you need to concentrate on increasing your intake of water as this will help you to get more energy and make you feel less hungry due to your tiredness.

Shift workers in particular have a difficult time in maintaining their weight because not only are they getting a lack of sleep but they will also be sleeping at various different times of the day and night and that affects your eating habits and your digestion.

Long-term lack of sleep will result in the body storing additional fat so it is essential to do all you can where possible to get a regular night's sleep at reasonable hours to maintain good health and a reasonable body fat percentage.

Obviously taking this to the other extreme where you are sleeping all hours of the day and not getting any exercise will also cause you to retain more body fat and increase weight.

Once again lifestyle has a huge bearing on whether you are at your optimum body weight or not.

Fad Diets Don't Really "Work"

It is not surprising that many people wonder why fad diets are bad when they seem to get results. You will find many infomercials on TV and online websites claiming significant weight loss in just a few days.

That type of weight loss is usually temporary. It is typically 90% water which will be put straight back on as soon as your body rehydrates. You'll need to rehydrate to maintain your health – and back comes the weight you supposedly "lost."

Other fad diets are not necessarily crash diets with outrageous claims. They are, more than likely, over-hyped diet plans that tend to be fashionable for a while and usually make a lot of money for the inventor.

In the best cases, these fad diets are good nutrition plans which will help you lose weight, but which you could probably have gotten for free from your doctor. In the worst cases, they will prove so difficult to follow that you will give up after a week. So much for sticking to a diet.

How Fad Diets Can Hurt You

1. Diets that promise quick and easy weight loss are usually based on eating more of one food type and none of another (e.g., grapefruits or cabbages). These do not give the benefits that you would get from a balanced diet.

They may suggest you take supplements but many supplements are not absorbed by the body unless they are taken along with the foods that the diet has banned. After a few weeks, if you stick to it that long, you may begin to develop nutritional deficiencies.

2. Fad diets are often boring and too restrictive. After the novelty of the first day or two, you will stop enjoying your meals.

You will then start to crave food constantly and will sooner or later (often sooner), break the diet. You may even feel guilty, thinking it is your fault that you did not lose weight.

3. Often the diet will recommend high fat foods and low carbs which, if taken long term, could result in heart disease. The research indicates that certain high fat foods such as foods with olive oil or fatty fish like sardines or wild salmon, may be good for you. But processed meats like deli meats, bacon, and sausages, can damage your health in the long run. So, finding a diet that tells you about good fats and bad fats can make a big difference.

The promoters of the average high fat diet should tell you that their diet is only intended to be followed for a short time. But you probably will not reach your goal weight in that time, and then what? You either continue with a plan that is not good for your health, or stop and probably gain back what you lost.

4. Many fad diets do not help you to incorporate enough servings of fruits and vegetables in your weight loss program, or give you the variety of foods that your body needs.

5. Quick weight loss diets are just a temporary solution and do not help you to make permanent changes to your eating habits. Permanent changes are the only way to remain at your target weight once you reach it.

Fad diets encourage yo-yo diet-binge cycles of fast weight loss and equally fast weight gain. This is worse for your health and your self esteem than if you had stayed over-weight all the time.

Whatever the publicity materials may say, these extreme diets will not help you in the long term. The best way to sustain weight loss is to eat a varied and healthy diet that avoids addictive trigger foods. Eat somewhat smaller portions, get active (stand up rather than sitting for hours) and exercise regularly. And, stay away from fad diets.

Your Action Steps:

1. Learn about the established diets that have healthy eating plans you can do. Decide what fits with your time and budget.

2. Check out the diet to make sure there are clear guidelines and recipe books to help you make a good menu and snack plan.

3. Modify the diet plan to accommodate avoiding the addictive foods you have identified in your tests for trigger foods.

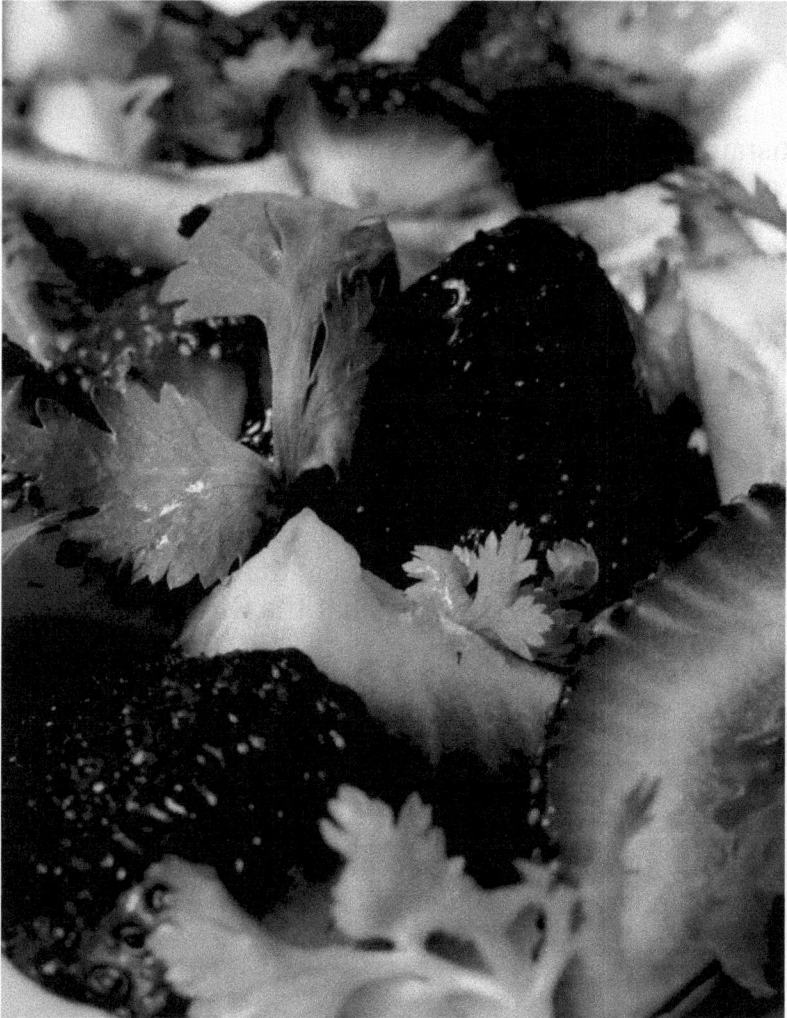

Motivational Strategies

"Do it, and then you will feel motivated to do it."

- Zig Ziglar

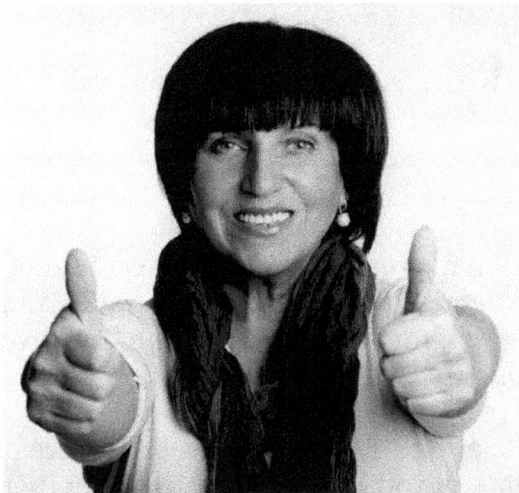

Part of sticking to a diet is finding the motivation inside yourself to persist.

When it comes to dieting, it also helps to understand what's driving your decision to lose weight. Sometimes it's not enough to be motivated to fit into a new dress.

Likewise the general desire to get healthy isn't always enough to keep you going.

You need to spell out exactly what it is you want to accomplish and why. Here are a few sample items that may motivate you:

- Look and feel great

- Reduce risk for heart disease

- Get off of medication for diabetes

- Live longer for your children or grandchildren

- Have fun shopping for clothes again

- Less pain in your joints

- Be able to move more easily

- Save your marriage

- Enjoy more activities such as gardening, walking, hiking, or traveling

Once you understand what's really motivating you to diet, you can write it down and place reminders around you. This will help you to focus on what you want to achieve whenever you're tempted to stray from your plan.

You can be very simple about it, or you can get very creative. Some people create vision boards to help remember goals and motivation. You can create this by simply putting magazine cutouts, photos, and even just words on a small poster.

This poster can very simple or more elaborate. When completed, place the vision board somewhere that you can look at it every day. Take a few moments each day and reconnect to your purpose and vision.

Other people create self-affirmations to place in prominent areas. For example, you may want to put small notes on your bathroom mirror, inside your car, and even on your desk at work.

These notes will serve as regular reminders that you have a greater purpose for sticking to your diet. Whenever you're feeling like you want to stop following the plan or you want to give up, you can go to these messages of motivation for inspiration.

Using rewards to reach a goal is not uncommon. It's done all the time in business as employers reward their employees with bonuses, trips and days off for a job well done. Retail stores motivate their customers to shop with them by offering discounts and loyalty cards you get punched each time you buy something there with the promise of something free the next time you go there. Find some way to reward yourself when you reach milestones along your way to your weight loss goal.

You may be familiar with the two types of motivation called Intrinsic and Extrinsic. Intrinsic motivation is when a person is motivated from within him or herself. They work on a task or project or to achieve a goal simply for the love of doing it. Extrinsic motivation is when a person works on a task or tries to reach a goal, but is rewarded when that goal or steps to that goal are reached.

Studies have shown that intrinsic is a better motivator than extrinsic but most of us are programmed to the point of not doing something unless we're rewarded. Mo-

49

tivation is a behavior you can influence to your advantage. It's important to realize that even a highly motivated person can get discouraged or tired of working on a task if she's not noticed and rewarded. People need to know they're appreciated and that their good work does not go unnoticed.

We're all different and motivated by different things. What motivates you may not motivate your spouse or your boss. It's a valued skill when you're able to match the type of motivation with the person to be motivated. Try different things and when one doesn't work try another until the desired results are accomplished.

Employers do this all the time but, unfortunately, many use fear motivation with the threat that you could lose your job if you don't do the work. This is not a permanent solution and most companies who implement this kind of motivation experience a high rate of employee turnover.

Begin with a realistic goal that is challenging and one that you'll feel a sense of pride when it's accomplished. If you're trying to lose weight, for instance, and your goal is to lose 10 pounds in 3 months, reward yourself for every milestone reached.

If you lost 3 pounds in the first month, celebrate by going to lunch with a friend or treat yourself to a pedicure. (Both men and women enjoy this.) Be happy with the reward and you'll start anticipating the loss of your next 3 or 4 pounds.

If you find it difficult to stick to the rules, work with a friend who will keep track of your progress and administer the reward when they're earned. Make the reward irresistible to you and make it worthwhile even though it doesn't have to be expensive. The experience you associate with the reward is what will keep you motivated.

Motivation rewards work for almost any desired goal and can work wonders with children. Remember to have your reward aligned with your goal and you're on the way to reaching your target with fun and anticipation.

Stress Relief Techniques – Not Junk Food

Stress-induced problems swirl around us all the time and it often feels like the pressure never ends! Yet, there are simple ways to relieve stress without harming your body.

With any mind-body technique or alternative therapy, you can benefit in multiple ways. The benefit is lowering your reactions to stress from everyday hassles that would otherwise trigger you to eat your comfort foods.

You know, comfort foods are not just "junk." Most can soothe you at a very basic biological and psychological level. It turns out that foods high in sugar and fats are comforting, even to animals distressed by being separated from their mother at an early age. People find these "high reward" foods comforting too.

The trouble is, "comfort foods" are often not so good for your health or your weight.

Here are 10 practical ways to relieve stress that don't involve grabbing a junk food or sugary snack for comfort.

10 Practical Stress Relieving Tips

Here are 10 ways to lower your stress:

1. **Cut out the busy-ness**. What are some things you can cut out of your schedule to give you more quality time for you and your family? Even giving yourself or your family 30 minutes a day makes a huge difference.

* What clubs or organizations do you belong to? What meetings or activities are you involved in? Is it all necessary?

* Carefully consider which programs and activities you can remove from your schedule - then do it! Saying "no" to others is like saying "yes" to yourself.

2. **De-clutter and organize your home**. When your home is cluttered and unorganized, you tend to feel cluttered and unorganized on the inside, causing you more stress.

* Get rid of the stuff you never use by selling it, throwing it away, or giving it to someone who'll make use of it. Once you've done that, organize what's left over and make a place for everything. If necessary, use labels and organizational containers to make it easy to find things again.

3. **De-clutter and organize your workspace**. Organizing your workspace is no different than de-cluttering your home.

* Remember, your external environment affects your internal peace. Messy on the outside likely means messy on the inside.

4. **One of the major stress factors is money. However, there's a simple solution: a budget.** Most people don't like the word budget, but budgeting doesn't have to be difficult. In fact, financial planning actually helps you save money.

* Do a search online to find a budgeting system that works best for you. It needs to be simple and easy to use every day. Once you're on a budget you'll feel a lot less stressed due to finances.

* Seek the help of an experienced financial planner who can steer you on the right financial path.

5. **Enjoy what you do have**. In our society you've probably learned somewhere along the way that more is better. Well, it's not.

* When you learn to be content with what you have right now, you'll find much more peace within yourself.

6. **Get regular exercise**. When you exercise, your body burns off more than just fat and calories. Working out also burns off steam.You feel better in many different ways.

* If you're stressed due to work situations or family conflict, getting a good workout will help you relieve stress. You'll be able to think and reason more clearly, which will help you deal with some of the core issues that are causing your stress.

7. **Eat healthier**. Yes, eating healthy foods really does relieve stress because when your body is nourished properly, it functions optimally. Eating right lends itself to clearer thinking.

8. **Reduce your workload**. If you have a heavy workload, either on the job or at home, do what you can to reduce it.

* Take a good look at your routine and determine if the workload is really worth the toll it's taking on your body and health. If it's not - and there's no end in sight - perhaps it's not the proper solution to your problems anyway.

9. **Communication is key to relieving stress in your life**. If you have a friend you can talk to openly and honestly, seek them out.

* Getting things off your chest will help you sort out problems and see your situation in a new light. The less foggy your mind is, the more stress you'll be able to remove from your life.

* It often helps to have someone outside of the situation to talk to because they'll likely see something you don't.

10. **Journaling is a great way to relieve stress**. You can have an outlet without having to reveal your deep thoughts to the rest of the world.

Get a special notebook to keep your journal writing in.

* Journaling is a great way to see the progress you've made, which can be very therapeutic.

This type of journal is focused more on writing down your feelings. You can and should also use your journal for recording more factual information about your diet, activity levels, and weight to track your progress.

As you can see, there are many ways to reduce stress. Put them into practice now and you'll soon begin to see a real difference in your life. Your stress will start to diminish and you'll be free to enjoy your beautiful life!

Meditation

Meditation is a way to promote overall well-being and improve your mental, emotional, and physical condition. Many different studies have shown that meditators cope better with stress — and stress is a common trigger for eating comfort foods that may taste good, but that contribute to weight gain in a big way.

If you are suffering from stress, meditation can be a great way to relieve the symptoms. Buddhist monks and nuns, who meditate often, are well known for being some of the calmest people on earth. Of course, meditation is practiced by Christians and people of many other religions too. Fortunately you can get a lot of the same benefits without checking in for life at the nearest monastery.

In order to relieve stress, meditation is usually practiced regularly. It is possible, of course, to sit down and meditate whenever you feel especially stressed, but often times this is not convenient. And you will get better results if you practice it often.

Try to meditate every day at the same time. For most people the best time is either first thing in the morning, last thing at night or after an exercise session.

Anti stress meditation does not have to be practiced for very long. It is much more effective to sit for 10 minutes, six days a week, than to meditate for a whole hour once a week.

Here are some simple steps to begin meditation:

- First make sure that you will not be interrupted during your meditation time. You might want to put a 'Do not disturb' notice on the door. Switch off your phone. Use some kind of timer or alarm so that you do not have to keep looking at a clock.

- Find a comfortable position either sitting or lying down. Lie flat on your back on the floor or on a mat, with no pillow. If you are sitting, you can be crosslegged on a cushion on the floor in the traditional meditation posture or use a chair. Be sure to keep your back straight. In a chair, have both feet flat on the ground.

- Be aware of your breath flowing in and out through your nostrils. You can either close your eyes or have them slightly open, looking down. You may find it helpful to work through the body, relaxing each part. Do not forget the muscles of the face, which carry a lot of tension.

- You will find that thoughts and emotions arise while you are doing this. Try to let them go. They will pass by themselves if you do not get caught up in them.

Some people find it helpful to listen to some relaxing music or sounds or water, birdsong etc while they meditate. There are many relaxation CDs that you can find in a music store or online.

It is better to get something that is specially designed for relaxation and does not include any lyrics. Songs can be very emotive and can arouse strong feelings, making you more stressed instead of less.

Alternatively, you might want to investigate binaural beats which play a special rhythm designed to set the brain's waves to a frequency that is associated with deep relaxation. You can play these on an MP3 player with stereo headphones. Just one warning: you may want to do this in the evening rather than earlier in the day, because binaural beats played during anti stress meditation can be so relaxing you will want to go to sleep right after you finish!

Visualization Techniques and Self Hypnosis

The surprising fact is that many conditions can be improved by visualization, which is a form of self hypnosis -- and weight loss is one of them. It works like this: you keep a vision in your mind of how you want your body to look, and subconsciously you will begin acting in a way that will go in that direction. You become much more positive about your body, more accepting of your diet or fitness regime, and you will reach your weight goals more quickly and easily.

Effecting change through visualizing desired outcomes has become more and more acceptable in recent years. Psychologists do not understand exactly how it works but clearly the mind and body are not as separate as we often believe. It seems that if you truly want something it is more likely to happen - provided of course that it is something that is possible, and within your control.

Visualization helps us to truly want to lose weight by creating a clear and happy picture of our fitter bodies. Without this we can often put psychological traps in our own path.

Many people who are overweight believe they cannot lose weight. Sometimes you may say it out loud, or hear friends say it about themselves. For other people this belief stays in the subconscious. But it is sure that it influences our behavior.

Someone who believes it is impossible for her to lose weight will be constantly battling her own negativity when she is trying to diet. Her mind will be constantly telling her there is no point dieting, she cannot lose weight so she should just go ahead and eat everything she wants. Visualization is the strongest technique that we can use to overcome these negative thoughts and impulses.

You can use self hypnosis to put positive ideas into your mind. These will reprogram how you think and feel -- allowing you to live in a more constructive and beneficial way.

If you are plagued by negativity either from your own mind or from the reactions of friends and family to your diet, go ahead and visualize yourself at your desired weight as often as you can. It works on the same level as all those negative voices and can annihilate their influence like nothing else can.

It is important to practice every day - morning and evening if you can. You just need to take a few minutes in a quiet place and keep an image in your mind of your body at its ideal weight.

Some people can do this easily, others need some help. If you have a photograph of yourself at your ideal weight in the past, you may find it easier to look at that. Or use a photo from a magazine but cut off the person's face. You need to visualize your own body, but thinner.

You can also visualize from the inside. Close your eyes and let your awareness focus on a part of your body - for example, your right thigh. Imagine it slowly becoming thinner in your mind's eye. Then move to the other thigh, and on through the body. It may help to start at the feet and move up towards the head, or vice versa.

As you go about your work or daily chores, think of yourself as already at your ideal weight. Create your own affirmations and repeat them often, always in the present tense ("I am glad to be flexible, fit and slim", not "I will ...").

Enjoy the feeling of having a positive self-image. Over time, this will help you to keep to your weight loss plan. You will find that fatty foods are less attractive and exercise is more enjoyable.

While your weight loss will of course be gradual, the wonderful thing about visualization is that it gives you a new body image right away. Use visualization and weight loss to make you happier right now, today!

Yoga

Most people have some form of addiction whether we like to admit it or not. For women with weight issues, the addiction likely involves specific foods.

For the most part we have a reasonable level of control over our addictions but they can be as minor as wanting to eat a little more chocolate than is healthy or they can be devastating – to binge on sweets daily and become massively obese. This level of overeating obviously creates other problems in our life.

It is difficult to eliminate the tendency toward addictions as many times it is due to something that has happened in the past. Many people can't even pinpoint what it might be that has caused the addiction. Food addiction may be even more primitive – based in the reward pathways of the brain for basic physical comfort.

So, what are your options?

Yoga is a spiritual, mental, emotional, and physical practice that began in ancient India. As with many such practices, you can use it for spiritual enlightenment, or you can use it just for promoting a better sense of well-being, inner balance, and peace.

Yoga helps to peel back the layers of time that have made us what we are and in that process we can begin to see the reasons why we have certain addictions.

People who are aware that they have an addiction often try to repress it, but this is not the way to solve the problem.

Yoga is even used in many drug and alcohol detox programs to help people come off drugs by recreating the balance in their life that they have lost along the way. Yoga helps people with physical symptoms like headaches or arthritis – problems that the trigger foods in food addictions can worsen.

By helping people to look at their way of thinking, that they have conditioned themselves to accept, yoga can help to make the necessary changes that will allow them to change their thought patterns and eliminate the addictive behavior faster than most other forms of help.

The major benefit of using yoga to assist in the treatment of addictions is the fact that it also helps people to change the way they feel about themselves.

Better self esteem flows over into all aspects of your life, giving you a more positive and productive approach to living.

Regular yoga practice will gently help you shift out of your compulsive eating binges and into an ability to stick with a diet.

Acupuncture

Acupuncture is a great way to relieve stress and strengthen your coping abilities. Stress is a natural part of life, but with our seemingly never-ending hectic lifestyles, we are more stressed out than ever!

This ancient healing art from China also has the ability to rebalance your system. Chinese medicine experts know a great deal about diet and can advise you on the types of foods that may work best for your particular body type and needs.

For instance, is it OK to eat cold foods – or do you need to eat warmer foods as much as possible. This will have implications for your ability to use a raw vegetable type of diet plan.

There are various techniques you can use to relieve stress, such as yoga, meditation, acupuncture, and more. You may want to try several methods of de-stressing to find a method you feel most comfortable with.

What is Acupuncture?

Acupuncture is an ancient Chinese healing art that involves inserting fine needles at very precise pressure points throughout the body. The needles stimulate the body's natural healing processes in its energy system.

How Does It Work?

Acupuncturists believe that energy flows through the body system through channels called meridians. This energy is referred to as Qi or Chi.

Stress causes an imbalance in the body's energy and causes it to flow improperly. The Qi can become blocked and stagnant. It must be unblocked and flow freely in order to restore harmonious balance to the body.

By stimulating the proper acupressure points, the Qi can flow freely, thereby alleviating stress induced mental and physical symptoms.

Is Acupuncture Safe?

Acupuncture is very safe when performed by a licensed practitioner. Acupuncturists are trained in the proper methods of treatment and all instruments are sterilized to prevent any risk of infection.

The Food and Drug Administration approved non-toxic disposable needles made for single use application just for use in acupuncture treatments. The majority of people who undergo acupuncture feel no pain at all. A small percentage may feel very minimal pain. Bleeding rarely occurs.

Don't let fear of needles stop you – there are forms of acupuncture that practitioners can do without any needles. Instead, they may use special laser light or micro-current stimulation of acupuncture points. You can look around in your local area for acupuncturists who offer these types of services.

Health Benefits

Acupuncture can relieve the physical symptoms of stress that tends to accumulate in the neck, shoulders, and back, causing pain and tension. Headaches are another physical complaint resulting from stress. People who are under high levels of stress often have high blood pressure.

Acupuncture can relieve physical symptoms, such as tense muscles, and even help to lower blood pressure. Acupuncture leaves the body feeling calm and relaxed. An added benefit of acupuncture is that it improves the circulation of the blood throughout the body. Certain protocols in acupuncture cut down on addictive cravings for foods or drugs.

Treatment Sessions

A typical acupuncture session may last for 30 to 60 minutes. The patient will become very relaxed during the treatment and may even fall asleep.

Regular acupuncture treatments can help strengthen your body so you're better able to deal with the day-to-day stresses of life. Acupuncture can also leave you feeling refreshed and energized.

Useful for Stress Related Health Conditions

Regular acupuncture treatments can help heal stress related health conditions and improve the body's immunity to defend against potential illnesses.

In fact, in some cases, acupuncture that is being used to treat one condition can actually help find or improve another, more severe illness that had not been previously identified. In such cases, acupuncture is part of early diagnosis and adjunctive treatment.

In another sense, acupuncture can serve as a form of preventive measure against illness by alleviating stress and strengthening the body.

The Mind-Body Connection

Acupuncture serves to the treat the mind and body as a whole system. Conventional medicine has come to accept that the mind affects the body. The mental system affects the physical. Stress is a perfect example of the interrelated connection between the body and mind.

The mind perceives life situations and the body reacts to them on the basis of the mind's perception. If the mind perceives a threat, the body immediately prepares for a flight or fight response in which the heart beats faster and the muscles tighten, just as with stress.

Remember, acupuncture is just one method of relieving stress. It's also important to learn positive and productive ways to cope with stress on a daily basis, thereby making the stress work for you rather than against you.

Find your own combination of de-stressing methods that work for you, and use them often to enjoy a happier and healthier life.

⟡

Your Action Steps:

1. Choose two motivation booster strategies to help you stay on your diet. Add these into your daily routine.

2. Select one of the alternative therapies (yoga, meditation, acupuncture) and find a local practitioner (or teacher, depending on the therapy). Make an appointment.

3. Find a self hypnosis audio recording that helps support you whenever you need a boost. Play it for yourself whenever it feels too hard to continue your diet plan.

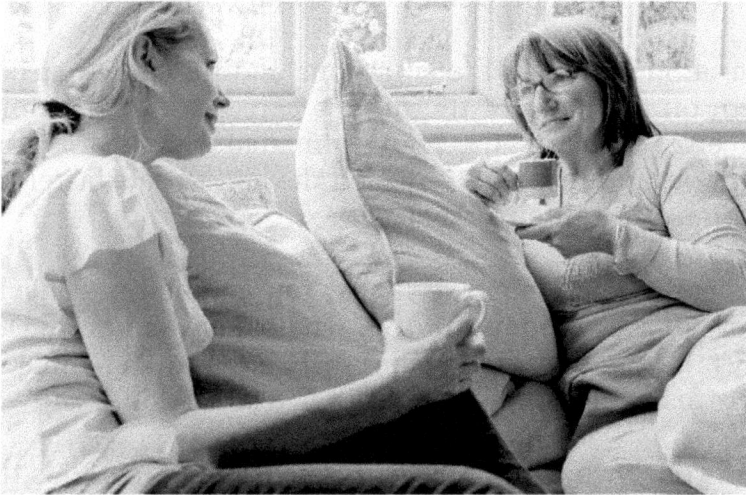

"A hero is an ordinary individual who finds the strength to persevere and endure in spite of overwhelming obstacles."

- Chrisopher Reeve

Successful Diet Planning for Women

"Plans are nothing; planning is everything."

- Dwight D. Eisenhower

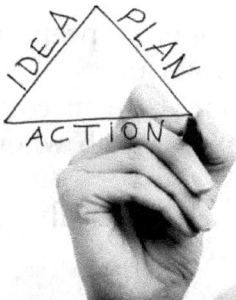

In order to stick to a diet, you need a good plan. To get a good plan, you have to do the planning.

Some of the tips for this planning may seem obvious and simple – but if you don't do them, you'll hit more challenges in staying on your weight loss and healthy eating program.

Planning What To Eat

When it's time to begin your healthy diet plan, it helps to make sure you have all the things you need to be successful. The key to successful planning is to know what you are going to eat and when you are going to eat it.

- Plan your weekly menu – many diet books will have 1-2 weeks' worth of sample menus for you to use

- Post your menu on the refrigerator so that you don't have to think about what to eat next

- Shop once a week for all of the items you will need in your menu

- Once you have done your food shopping, prepare as much of the food in advance as you can
  - Cut up your veggies and put them in containers so that they are easy to grab when you want a snack
  - Pre-cook protein sources that can easily be re-heated in a microwave oven

- Be prepared for the unexpected – keep a bag of nuts in your purse or briefcase, take an apple or other piece of allowed fruit with you when you are out of the house, bring along a piece of cheese (if allowed on your diet plan)

Some diet plans have staple items that you'll need over and over again. You may find that it's best to buy these items in bulk so that you get a better bargain. When you buy in bulk, you'll also have more on hand.

You also want to be sure and stock supplies such as storage containers, plastic wrap, and aluminum foil that you'll need if you're cooking for yourself a lot. Some diets also require supplements and you'll need to have a large supply of them.

If you're using prepackaged food, it's important to have a good stock on hand so that you don't have an emergency. When you run out of your pre-packaged food, you'll have to make something different.

If things really go wrong with your weekly menu, make sure you're prepared with a backup menu that does not throw you off your diet.

There are some diets that require special equipment such as a blender or a microwave. Make sure you have these items before you begin a diet that requires them. Having supplies ahead of time will help you stick to your diet.

If you're going to make exercise a part of your program, you'll also want to make sure you've got the appropriate clothing and footwear. You don't want to find that you don't have comfortable shoes when you're a few days into the program. Get your gym membership set up if you want to do your exercise there.

Before you start your diet you need to make a checklist of the things you'll need. Keep this checklist handy so that you'll always know what you need to buy – even if you have to make a quick run to the store after work.

Once you've got all the supplies you need, you'll be prepared to stick with your diet for the long term. When you're not prepared, it makes it that much easier to slip up and miss your routine.

Find Your Support Group

Local or Online Weight Loss Support Groups

When it comes to dieting, it's often better not to go it alone. It often helps to have someone to whom you can be accountable. It's also nice to have someone who shares your common goals and vision.

You may want to consider starting a diet group or even just having a diet buddy. This person will help you to stay on track and you will do the same for him or her. When you work together, you have several benefits:

• You can share success stories

• You can share obstacles and brainstorm ideas to overcome them

• You'll be able to swap recipes

• You'll have accountability (check in with one another for a few minutes every day)

• You can motivate one another

• Together you can focus when other areas of your life distract you from taking care of yourself

70

When it comes to finding the right type of support, there are a few things to keep in mind. First, you'll want to find someone who is positive about the process and who is committed.

If you work with someone who's not really committed, you may find that you spend all of your energy trying to stay focused while they distract you. You'll want to talk before you partner up and find out how committed they are to the process.

You'll also need to look for someone who has a similar schedule and will be available at about the same time you're available. This way you know that you'll be able to meet consistently.

In addition, you probably want to find someone who is following the same diet that you're following. This way you can truly share stories and you can brainstorm ways to get through stumbling blocks.

Having that support you need can be critical to your success. It's possible to do it on your own, but it's so much easier when you have someone to share the burden of this major lifestyle change.

Once you've found someone to work with you, make sure that you are also committed to the process. Be his or her cheerleader and follow through will all of your promises when it comes to meeting and working together.

Steer Clear of the Doubters

Just as you need support from other people to stick with your diet, you also need to stay away from people who seem to want you to fail. It's a well known fact that when you're trying to lose weight and improve your health, someone will come along to sabotage your efforts.

Whether it's jealousy, misunderstanding, low self-esteem on their part, sympathy for your "deprived" state, or just plain being mean, this is something you should expect.

There are several ways you can handle the doubters in your life:

• If possible, avoid them altogether – this is difficult if it's a close friend or family member

• When you are together, avoid talking about the subject of dieting and weight loss – don't let them in on your diet plan

• Or, confront the person and let them know you won't be discussing your diet with them and you would like them to please stop any behaviors that are getting in your way

• Whatever they do or say, ignore their efforts to defeat you diet – don't engage them when they try to stop your progress

Efforts of other people to get in the way of your success are a sad truth when it comes to dieting. There will always be people who – consciously or unconsciously – will try to keep you from making things work.

Sometimes it's enough to just recognize that this is happening so you can avoid them or confront them on the issue. While having positive support can lead to your success, allowing negative people to get in your way will be detrimental.

It's best to nip the problem in the bud. The first time someone does or says something that makes your diet more difficult, make sure to let them know what you want from them.

Change is a hard pill to swallow. Some people – even people who care about you – will have a hard time if your new lifestyle interferes with theirs. Remember that we don't live in a bubble. Our actions always affect others.

For example, if they're used to going out to dinner or dessert, it may be difficult when you either turn them down or don't eat that brownie a la mode anymore. This is especially true if he or she needs to lose weight as well.

But most people will get over their problems and turn into supporters if you make it clear that you're committed to your new plan. And eventually as you succeed, they'll cheer you on.

Journals Can Help You with Your Weight Loss Plan

Study after study has found that the most successful dieters are those who keep a journal. This journal can work in a number of ways and you can tailor the process to the particular diet you've chosen.

For some people, keeping a journal will mean writing down calories and fat grams. For other people it will mean writing down the specific foods and portions you enjoy at each meal.

And, to help reduce stress, record how you feel about things going on in your daily life, your eating, your diet, and your progress.

Still for others, it will mean keeping track of when you ate and how you felt at the time. Some journals are for keeping track of emotions and hunger. But no matter what you do, it helps to keep a journal to record the process.

In addition to keeping track of your diet in your journal, you can also use it to track the amount of exercise you complete. You can also track your weight and inches in the journal to have all the important information in one place.

Your journal can be something you purchase directly from your diet program. It may also be something that you simply purchase at the office supply store. A spiral notebook often works very well and is an inexpensive choice.

If you need to keep your journal with you on the go, then you'll want to purchase a very small book that can fit in your pocket, briefcase, glove box, or purse. In that case you may also want something that has a sturdy cover to handle wear and tear.

Journals can be very versatile and fit your personal style. But the main thing you need to remember is that once you've bought the perfect book, you need to actually write in it. A journal that you don't use is worthless.

Here are a few tips for using your journal consistently:

•   Keep your journal on the kitchen counter where you normally prepare and eat food

•   If you eat out or travel a lot, keep a small journal that you can take with you

•   Journal your food in the morning when you plan your meals. At night you can go back and change anything that you did differently

•   Keep a pen or pencil attached to your journal

•   Write down what you ate – whether it was on your diet or not

•   Look back at your journal to find what weeks you were most successful, then simply repeat them

•   Use your journal to make a grocery list

A journal will make a huge impact on how well you stick to your diet. It offers built-in motivation for your journey. You'll have it to write in when you're not so happy about dieting and also when you have successes.

Your Action Steps:

1. Decide if you want a local support group, an online support group, or just a buddy.

2. Make the calls, join the group, set up the buddy appointment

3. Get a journal in which you can keep you food record easily. Record not only what you eat, but how it makes you feel and how it affected your weight.

4. Weigh yourself daily or at least weekly.

Experts differ on how often to do this – but they have found that getting feedback on any weight loss or habit change progress helps people stick with the plan and increase their chances of success.

Setting Healthy Weight Loss Goals

"If what you are doing is not moving you towards your goals, then it's moving you away from your goals."

- Brian Tracy

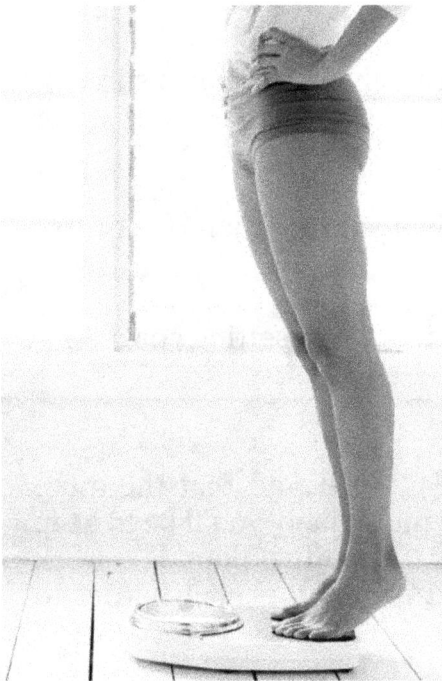

Setting healthy weight loss goals is another key to your success in sticking to your diet.

A big stumbling block that many women face when dieting is setting unrealistic goals.

This creates a cycle that makes it difficult to stay on your diet. What often happens is that people become discouraged when they don't reach their goals. This discouragement eventually leads to giving up on the diet.

But instead of giving up, most people would benefit more from actually being more realistic about their expectations.

From the beginning you need to make sure you set goals you can actually achieve. This helps to build success and motivate you to continue further. Slow and steady wins the race.

✧

Here are a few things to consider when setting goals:

•   Weight goals should be reasonable – 1-2 pounds per week

•   Goals having to do with behavior are also successful. For example, set a goal to drink 8 glasses of water each day for a week.

•   You shouldn't try to change more than one or two behaviors at a time.

•   Don't compete with others when setting goals.

As you go about setting goals, you'll find that the more small successes you have, the more likely you'll be to keep going. Many people who try to lose five pounds a week find that they can't do it and it only makes it harder to keep going.

Your goals need to be very specific and very measurable. To have the goal to "lose weight" isn't enough. You must set smaller goals such as losing 1 pound per week for 52 weeks. This is very specific and each week you can check in to see if you met your goal.

When you make goals that are too large or too vague, you set yourself up for failure. You'll have a problem before you even begin your work. Don't set yourself up for failure by being to broad with your goal setting.

Most successful people find that setting goals is one of the most important parts of achieving those goals and this applies to almost everything in life including your ability to be successful with weight loss.

What you do have to realize however is these goals need to be realistic and you need to believe that you can achieve them or you will be starting off on the wrong foot and failure will be imminent.

To make your goal achievable you need to look at it over an extended period of time rather than believing that you can lose 15 pounds in a couple of weeks.

While this might be possible it is certainly a lot harder to achieve than to expect to lose that weight over the course of several months.

Keeping a journal helps a lot of people to achieve their goals as it helps to enforce the actions that are required to meet those goals on a daily basis.

In your journal you can record your body weight, the foods you've been eating, any supplements you have been taking and the results that you have been getting from these actions. Write down how you feel about your progress as well.

This helps you to readjust your goals and make changes to your fitness and nutrition as things change in the course of your weight loss program.

Within your major goal you should also have short-term goals and once again these need to be realistic to keep you motivated.

These short-term goals will change from time to time. During the course of your weight loss program, you will probably find that progress accelerates after certain stages of your plan.

Sometimes you will also plateau for a while where your weight loss will tend to slow down. By having a journal, you will be able to look at those areas that you might be able to change to get over that plateau and continue with your progress.

Creating Your Weight Loss Progress Chart

Keeping a journal and making goals are great first steps for getting your diet in gear. But you also want to make sure you chart your progress as you diet so that you can see both your successes and your failures.

Charts and graphs offer visual representations of your progress. You can make a line graph of your weight loss in pounds and in inches. You can also make graphs that show your goals and your achievements.

When you see your success visually, it can be a huge motivator to keep going. And when you see the line on your graph start to veer off course, you can avoid further detours by kicking things back into gear.

Many people who have achieved dieting success have found charts and graphs to be critical to that achievement. You'll likely find that you have the same results when you begin to make graphic representations.

You can make charts by hand. And if you're comfortable with spreadsheets, you can plug the numbers in and let the computer do all the designing. Then you'll have it stored and you can manipulate the data to make the kind of graph you want.

Adapting Your Goals

You've been plugging along and your diet started out okay, but now you're finding that it doesn't fit your life-style or your budget well. Don't let this be a reason to give up or quit. This is just a time to reevaluate.

Sometimes you need to make changes in order to continue with your success. You may find that one diet may not work very well, but you can try a new program to keep going with your progress.

81

Every month or so, you'll want to ask a few questions about your diet:

- What have my successes been?

- Can I afford this program?

- Do I have enough time to follow this diet?

- Do I enjoy the food I am eating?

- Do I have more energy than I had before?

- Am I happy on this diet?

- Can this diet work for me long-term?

- Is there another diet that would work better for me?

If you're finding that you don't have energy, you're always hungry, and/or you hate what you're eating, it may be time for a change. Even if you're losing weight, you don't want to be miserable all the time.

Likewise, you may be feeling okay with the diet, but not losing any weight. If this is happening, you may need to find something that's more appropriate for you. However, if you're losing 1-2 pounds per week you're on target.

Sometimes people get discouraged because they want to lose 5 pounds every time they step on the scale. But you need to go back and remember to set realistic goals. A diet that causes more rapid weight loss may not be healthy.

If you find it's time for a change, don't hesitate to do what will make you more successful. Look for another program that works for you. Maybe one that fits your budget, schedule, or food preferences better.

There are hundreds of diets on the market and there's no reason to stick with something that isn't working for you. It may take five or six tries to discover what really works for you. The key here is to not give up.

Your Action Steps:

1. Set your weight loss goals week by week.

2. Get a little monthly calendar book to keep notes on your progress.

3. Review your progress each month and go over the questions in this chapter on what you think about how it is going.

Don't judge yourself – judge the diet plan.

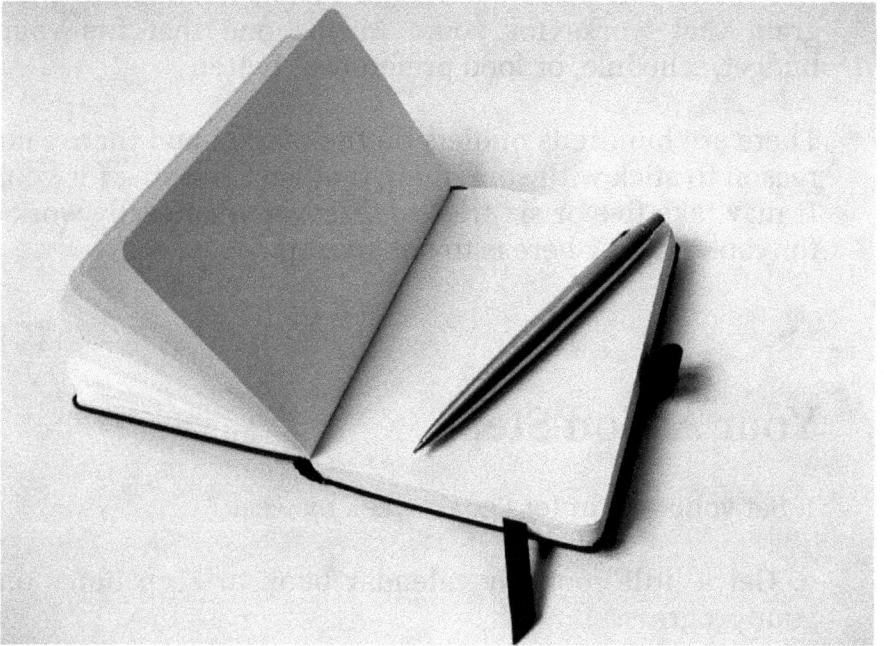

How To Be on a Diet and a Budget

"Some couples go over their budgets carefully every month. Others just go over them."

- Katherine Mansfield

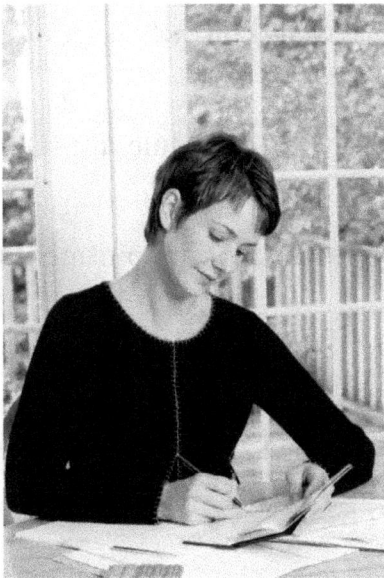

Weight loss does change the reality of your finances. In today's economy, many people are working to make sure they don't overspend.

Dieting is one of the places where people spend the most money. But it is possible to diet without overspending.

There are two routes you can take to dieting success when it comes to your budget. You can join a program that has costs attached to it or you can do it on your own and use a program from a book or other source.

Diet programs that offer fee-based services have benefits and drawbacks:

•   Often program fees are high and don't cover the cost of food

•   Even a diet that comes with prepackaged food must be supplemented with more food

•   You may get personal one-on-one service

•   You may get support group meetings

•   You have accountability and regular weigh-ins

•   You have someone to coach you when you're struggling and celebrate your successes

•   You must make time in your schedule for any regular appointments or classes

•   You may have to pay for meetings or appointments even if you don't attend them

Budget and personal preferences may make you prefer to handle the whole process yourself. That is fine too.

If you choose the option of going on your own, you'll find that there are also benefits and drawbacks:

•   You can use information from books, magazines, or online resources to tailor a plan for you – many of these sources are inexpensive or free

•   You won't have as much accountability

•   You won't have to buy expensive prepackaged food, but you will have to spend more time preparing food

•   Support can be encouraged by working with friends, but you won't have a built-in coach

•   You won't have to schedule regular appointments or meetings

Ultimately, as we keep saying in this book, you need to choose a diet you can stick with in the first place. If you're choosing something that's way out of your budget, you won't be able to afford it long-term. It's important that you make wise financial decisions early on in the process.

Setting up a diet that you will continue after the early enthusiasm might wane a bit is important. Chances are, buying prepared foods for your meals is not going to be your best choice. You are likely to want to prepare your own meals going forward.

Grocery Shopping on a Budget

Most women on a diet need to buy foods that they might not usually choose at the grocery store. Many times, those foods will cost more than some mass produced processed junk food. So, your goal is to get the goods without straying from the amount of money you have in your budget for buying food.

If you're a frequent grocery shopper you're aware of the constant increase in food prices. We all must eat so not shopping is not an option. Play the grocery game and develop a strategy to save as much as possible.

But, it's more than clipping coupons. It takes hard work and planning. Make a list and stick to it. Check to see what you already have so you don't come home with duplicate items that may go to waste.

Shop alone if you have discipline. Those extra helpers, be they children or spouse, can add extra goodies to the basket that are not needed -- and not on your well thought out list.

Don't shop on an empty stomach, especially when you are on a diet. If you do, everything looks good and you'll find yourself straying from the list. You might want to have a small allowed snack before you shop to curb any ravenous appetite.

Compare the unit price and buy a larger size if it's less per ounce or per pound. You can always divide it up in smaller packages when you get home. Higher priced items are usually placed at eye level so look up or down for lower priced foods. More expensive items are also usually on the high traffic aisles so wander off the beaten path.

Do your own slicing and dicing. Those prepackaged meats and cheeses are convenient but it is worth the price? Bulk cheese is cheaper and said to be healthier. Buying a whole chicken is much cheaper.

Cut it into parts later. Freeze what you don't need right away. Less tender cuts of meat are cheaper and if prepared right can be just as delicious.

The same goes for cereal. Those tiny one person servings cost more so buy the larger boxes. Hot cereals are usually less expensive per serving than the ready to eat cereal.

Bake from scratch. Need gluten free foods? You have many excellent options these days, from rice pasta to gluten free flours, to make meals that are on your tolerated food list. Read labels very carefully.

You pay more for ready mixes of cakes and cookies. Prepared foods will cost you more so do a little more work and save. Even the fancy cut pastas, rather than the plain, will add to your grocery bill.

Look for the mark down areas. You might find fresh meat or vegetables that are about to go out of date but if you're cooking them soon and freezing them, that's no problem. In fact, cooking some of the foods allowed on your diet in advance will make it easier to pop them into the microwave and have what you need fast for a meal when you are in a hurry.

Check the receipt for errors. Stores don't do this intentionally but it happens frequently. It could be entered incorrectly on the computer scanner or the checker could be rushed and enter the wrong amount purchased.

Check for errors as soon as you can and don't be shy about getting it corrected. Most stores are apologetic and give you a cheerful refund.

Plan a shopping day and avoid unnecessary trips. Keep your recipes simple and shop happy. Angry shoppers tend to impulse buy. Shop early and avoid the frantic crowds. Some consider grocery shopping good therapy while anticipating those delicious and healthy meals for themselves and family.

It's all in your attitude and your actions.

Your Action Steps:

1. Eat a meal or snack of permitted foods from your diet before you go grocery shopping.

2. Scan online and in the newspapers for local coupons and ads for bargains that fit into your diet. Ignore "bargains" that are not allowed on your diet.

3. Make your grocery shopping list and a checklist of steps to take from this chapter *before* you go to the store.

Stick with your list so that you can stick to your diet and your budget.

Exercise and Weight Loss

"Walking is the best possible exercise.
Habituate yourself to walk very fast."

- Thomas Jefferson

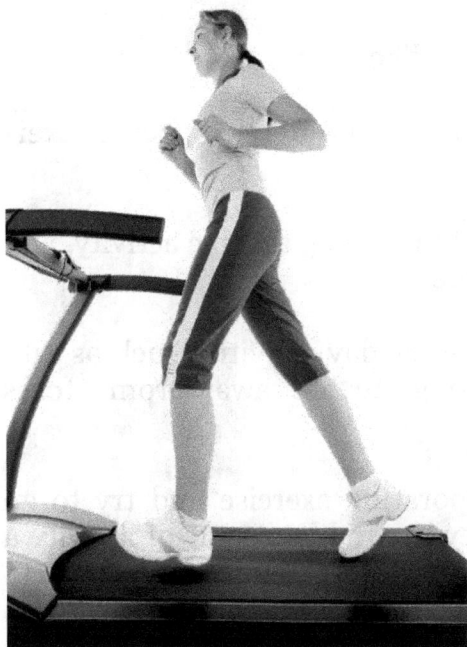

Exercise...

The dreaded activity that every doctor and health professional asks you to consider.

If you're looking for a way to boost the effects of your diet, you can't find anything better than exercise.

It can mean the difference between success and failure – sticking with a diet or not, for many women.

Yes, this does take work, and it isn't always easy. But if you add even a little exercise to your diet program you'll find that you exponentially increase your success.

Here are a few tips for adding exercise into your day.

•	Start slow – don't begin exercising and expect to win a marathon

•	Add 10 minutes of exercise into your day at first, then work up from there

•	Find a workout buddy who will go with you to exercise

•	Choose exercises you like

•	Change your routine – do different types of exercise regularly

•	Incorporate strength training, aerobic activity, and stretching into your routine

•	Add exercise into every day activities such as taking the stairs and parking further away from stores entrances

Many people start incorporating exercise and try to go way too fast at first. They may add an hour of activity a day – but after a few days that turns out to be too much. Instead, you'll want to start out slow.

Just adding 10 minutes a day will allow you to have improvement. And if you do 10 minutes for a week or two, you can add five more at a time. You want to be in this for the long run.

Also, think about the kinds of exercises you like to do. For some people there's no such thing as good exercise. But you may find that there are activities that will get your body moving without making you miserable.

Here are a few examples:

- Swimming

- Walking

- Bicycling

- Rollerblading

- Dancing

- Belly dancing

- Yoga

- Badminton

- Golf

- Fishing

- Gardening

- Hiking

- Cross country skiing

- Skiing

- Water skiing

- Flying a kite

- Frisbee

- Racquetball

- Squash

- Team sports

- Circuit training

- Weight lifting

And, no matter what, just walking regularly is great exercise and studies have shown it to be a great health boosting part of a total plan.

Walking is something you can do by yourself, with a buddy, or with your dog. You can find a local mall to walk if the weather is too cold, rainy, or snowy. Explore the neighborhood, or use a treadmill at home or in a gym.

Just get moving, somehow.

No matter what activity you try, exercise can be fun and make you feel better than just about anything. It helps you to produce natural hormones called endorphins that lift depression and give you huge amounts of energy.

If you're charting your progress, pay attention to what happens when you add even a tiny amount of exercise. You'll find that you have much greater success than you were having before.

One thing you need to know, though, is that you might actually see a small increase on the scale when you begin exercising – this is actually a good thing. If you've been extremely sedentary you're going to begin adding muscle mass to your body.

This muscle mass is lean tissue that's very compact. It will make you look leaner and you'll see your inches decreasing even if your weight goes up a pound or two. Eventually, the muscle tissue will help to raise your metabolism.

When that happens, you'll find that you lose weight faster, can eat more calories, and have more energy than you've had in the past. The benefits of exercise also extend to your health. Exercise will help you to enjoy:

• Lower risk of heart disease

• Lower risk of diabetes (and in some cases a reversal of it)

• Lower risk of cancer

• Lower risk of stroke

• Lower risk of arthritis

• Increased focus

- Increased energy

- Ability to move easily

- Decreased aches and pains

No pill on the market can give you all of these benefits. And while you'll have to get disciplined and into a new routine, you'll find that you never made a better decision in your life.

Many people believe that if they start exercising they will become hungrier and tend to eat more and fear that they will put on weight due to the fact that they will be consuming more food.

What they don't realize is the fact that your blood sugar levels determine when you feel hungry. When your blood sugar drops you will begin to feel hungry and seek food to increase the level again.

Exercising helps to normalize fluctuations in your blood sugar levels and in doing so you won't get that starving feeling as often.

Exercise activates your muscles which in turn burns fat rather than carbohydrates so this reduction in the burning of carbohydrates maintains your blood sugar levels in a more balanced manner.

By raising your metabolic rate from exercise the cells of your body will burn oxygen more efficiently and that in turn helps you to use the nutrients from your diet more effectively. It also helps to eliminate waste products and in doing so you are getting better nourishment from the foods that you eat.

By getting more nourishment you don't require the same quantities of food to feel satiated and fulfilled.

Another benefit of exercise is the fact that you are increasing your body temperature. This will help to mobilize the fat in your body that is used for energy rather than food. Your resting basal metabolic rate will also be raised after exercise for a considerable amount of time. Bottom line - exercise effectively helps you to burn more fat and improve the ratio of body fat percentage in your body.

There are so many positive reasons why you should be including some form of exercise into any weight-loss program and even if you are reluctant to exercise you should understand that it is probably easier to increase the exercise than to reduce the amount of food that you feel like eating every hour of the day.

Your Action Steps:

1. Talk with your doctor about what level of activity or exercise is the right way for you to start.

2. Come up with a plan to include regular activity in your daily routine. Get yourself a pedometer to tell you your progress in the number of steps you take each day.

3. Start with regular walking and build up from there. Remember to do the right stretching and preparatory moves before you exercise to keep down the risk of injury from being just a "weekend warrior."

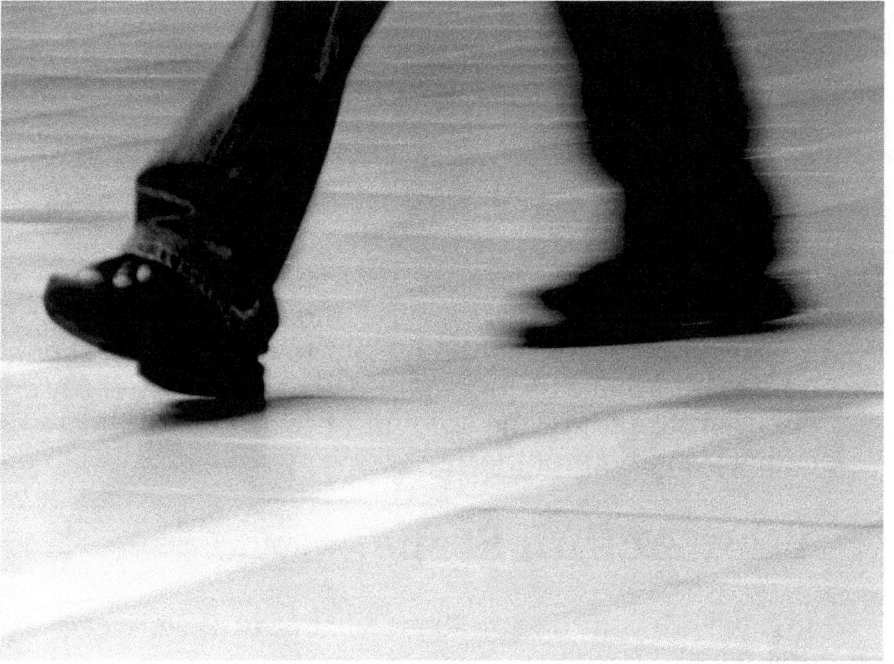

Tips for Enjoying Your Progress & Dealing with Setbacks

"Defeat is not the worst of failures. Not to have tried is the true failure." - George Edward Woodberry

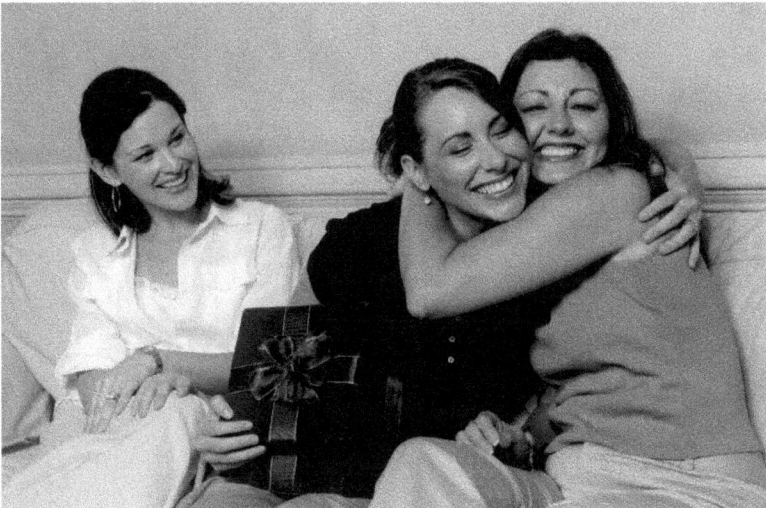

To be realistic, you are going to have good moments and bad ones on your way to weight loss and a healthy eating lifestyle. Here are some pointers for making your journey a lot easier.

Reward Yourself for Progress

When you get a new job, win a competition, or finish an important project, you probably reward yourself. When it comes to dieting, you'll want to do the same. If you've done something well, you'll want to pat yourself on the back.

If you're dieting in the first place, you may have once used food as a reward. This is no longer the best way to reward your achievement. Instead, you'll want to look at non-food rewards to celebrate. For example:

- Get a massage

- Enjoy a manicure and pedicure

- Buy a new outfit

- Go on a mini-vacation

- Take a bubble bath

- Go dancing

- Play a round of golf

- Go to a concert or other type of performance

- Have a movie night or even a special theater night

- Tell your support group and let them reward you

- Buy flowers for yourself

These are little treats that you can enjoy that help to make success a little sweeter. You don't have to spend a lot of money to enjoy something special. Sometimes locking yourself in your bedroom and letting your husband take care of the kids is treat enough.

But when you allow yourself to celebrate successes, you'll feel renewed. That will help you to stick to your diet and get to your next celebration. You may want to celebrate at a specific weight milestone.

But you may also want to celebrate successes in changing your behavior. For example, celebrate the first week you drank 8 glasses of water every day. That's something totally within your control – while the numbers on the scale are not.

What To Do When You Fall Off the Wagon

From time to time, you're going to go off of your plan. You may have an extra slice of cake, go carb crazy, or simply throw out all the rules for a vacation. It's okay to forgive yourself and move on when this happens.

The danger is when you beat yourself up, decide that you can't do it, and then throw out the diet completely. No one is perfect. If you were perfect, you would not need a weight loss plan. But, you are human. That's just fine.

Accepting that sometimes you'll make mistakes is a healthy way to stick to your diet in the long run.

Just regroup and keep going. The very next day you can pick up where you left off and pretend that you never went off course. Don't let a little setback actually throw you completely off of your diet.

Don't beat yourself up when you make mistakes with your diet. When you get discouraged, you may turn to food for comfort. This will cause you to stay off of your diet longer, gain weight, and feel even more discouraged.

This cycle is what causes people to gain weight quickly when they quit a diet program. You don't have to quit just because you made some mistakes. You just need to get back into the program.

You can also try to determine what caused you to go off track in the first place. This can help you to prevent future problems. Make your mistakes learning experiences and you'll have even more success.

Review Your Goals and Progress

Chances are that this isn't your first time to go on a diet. You may have tried over and over again only to experience failure. But this time you're ready to stick to your diet and achieve your goals.

It sometimes helps to look back at what caused you to get off course in the first place. You could have allowed discouragement to allow you to quit. You may have had a major life changing event that took you off the diet.

You may have chosen diets that didn't work for you financially or fit into your schedule. It's possible that your diet left you feeling so deprived that you would binge every few days.

Think back on all of your past experiences and determine what it is that caused you to fail. Then try not to repeat those same mistakes. This is one of the easiest ways to stick to your diet.

If you continue to do the things that didn't work for you in the past, you'll continue to have the same disappointments. Make this time different. Make this the time that you find a diet that's realistic for you and achieve success.

Your Diet and Your Family

It's really difficult to stick to a diet plan when you're the only one in your household doing it. If your family sits down to a big meal every night and you're the only one eating a "diet" meal, you'll fee very isolated.

By getting the whole family involved, you'll find that you achieve more success. You'll also be helping your whole family to improve their eating habits and their health. If you've had trouble with your weight, they may have the same problem.

While you may not call it a "diet" you'll find that your family probably needs to improve their eating habits as well. And it's extremely beneficial for your children to develop healthy eating habits that will follow them into adulthood.

Here are a few tips for getting the whole family involved in healthy eating:

• Prepare nutritious meals every night

• Eat together as a family

• Allow your children to help plan menus and cook food

• Serve at least 2 vegetables with every meal

• Only serve 1 starch at any meal

• Make sure you have protein with every meal

• Work with your children to pack healthy lunches instead of eating cafeteria food

• Don't make your child clean his or her plate – let them stop eating when they're satisfied

• Have fruit with meals as a substitute for sugary desserts

• Have a family activity night – go to the park, play in the yard, or take a walk together

• Limit video games to 1 hour a day

• Turn off the TV and play games with your family

• Eat breakfast together in the mornings

It would definitely be easier to hit the drive thru every night and then veg out in front of the TV. But when you take the extra time to make your whole family a part of it, you'll improve everyone's health.

In addition to the physical health benefit, you'll also grow closer as a family when you work together to create meals and have fun playing together. Your family will be both healthier and happier.

Restaurant Eating on a Diet

One of the biggest difficulties people have with dieting is figuring out what to do when eating out. Some people quit their diet altogether because they can't stick to it with their busy schedule.

But you can eat out and stick to your diet – if you choose the right diet in the first place. It just take a little plan-ning ahead to make sure you get the food you need to stay on your plan.

Here are a few tips for eating out at a sit-down restaurant:

•   Call ahead and have a menu faxed to you

•   Decide what you'll eat before you get to the restau-rant

•   Look on the menu for healthier selections – many restaurants have special diet menus

- Choose grilled food over fried food

- Ask for steamed vegetables

- Skip the bread basket

- Resist the urge to eat everything on your plate – stop when you're satisfied

- Split a meal with someone else

- Opt for water to drink with your meal

- If you have dessert, choose a small serving if on the menu or split it

- Choose whole grain pasta and bread if available

People are more health-conscious when it comes to eating out these days. Most major restaurant chains have developed menus for lighter fare. You can use these to help you make choices without having to think too much.

If you're on the go and you spend a lot of time eating fast food, you'll need to be prepared to choose healthy options. Here are some tips for fast food restaurants when you're on a diet:

- Get grilled food instead of fried food

- Drink diet sodas or water with your meal

- Ask for a side salad or fruit instead of fries

- Ask for food to be prepared without dressings, you can add your own instead

- Choose smaller portions – don't super size

- Try getting a kids meal

When you plan ahead for fast food, you can eat on the go and still stick to your diet. Most fast food restaurants now have choices for people who are trying to watch their weight or health.

Going to a Party

Another situation you may encounter is attending a party.

Many people fear that they won't be able to attend parties that are focused on food. But there are ways to survive when you attend a party. For example:

- Offer to bring a dish that is on your diet

- Eat before you go to the party so that you're not starving when you get there

- Look for items such as fresh veggies and fruits

- Eat small portions of higher calorie foods

- Drink water instead of sodas or mixed drinks

- Skip the cake – or have half a slice

- Don't fast all day and then binge at the party – eat your regular meals so that you don't overindulge

- Focus on friendships and socializing rather than food

Parties don't have to be miserable experiences where you feel deprived and unable to participate. And you don't have to skip them altogether. Just plan ahead so that you can make healthy choices.

Eating Lunch at Work on a Diet

Work lunches and break rooms can also be places where you can struggle with your diet. It helps to pack your lunch every day. Not only will you save money, but you won't be tempted to eat high calorie foods that aren't on your plan.

When it comes to the break room, you can't blame others for your problems with food. Instead of complaining about the lunch goodies that are brought, bring healthy alternatives. Celery or carrots with peanut or almond butter are healthier than any "energy" bar – and cheaper.

You can also keep plenty of healthy snacks at your desk to get through times of hunger. This will help you to resist the cakes, cookies, and breads that often are brought to the workplace.

Avoid Letting the Diet Become a Stressor for You

When you're on a diet, sometimes things won't go your way. You may plan ahead but find that a restaurant or party simply doesn't have what you need to stick to your plan. You may go to a friend's for dinner and not find any healthy selections on the menu.

If you're too rigid about your diet, you'll isolate yourself and alienate your friends. There will be times that you have to just go with the flow and be a little bit more flexible. If you do, you'll find that your diet will be more successful.

When you find yourself in a situation where you can't find diet-friendly foods, just use your common sense. Eat smaller portions, make the best choices you can, and get back on track when you return to a situation you can control.

When you're too rigid, it causes you to become discouraged. And when life throws something unexpected at you, you get completely off track. By staying flexible, you'll always be able to deal with changes.

And, if it does get to you, go back and review the options you have for managing stress that we discussed earlier in the book. Those strategies can make a big difference for you.

The Long-Term View

Take the longer term view. If you look at going on a diet as a temporary situation, you may have harder time sticking to it. Instead, you need to look at your diet as a lifestyle change. Instead of "going on a diet" you're changing your diet.

When you think of a diet as something that has an end, you set yourself up for weight gain and discouragement. You'll have to maintain a healthy lifestyle in order to enjoy the success you've achieved.

Sometimes just making this simple change in the way you view your situation will help you to have more short-term success. It can also help you to have long-term success and the results you really want.

Your Action Steps:

1. **Choose the reward** that you will give yourself when you achieve your first milestone of the diet plan.

Draw a picture or find a picture and post it in a place you see every day (on your refrigerator or over your desk or on the corner of your bathroom mirror).

2. **Practice what you will say and do** if a family member or friend expresses doubt or says negative things about your diet or your progress on the diet.

Make notes on your best responses to these scenarios.

3. **Make a list of the situations that you anticipate** will come up when you are needing to have meals out of your home (restaurants, work lunches, parties, etc)

Write down the diet options you will have if dealing with each of the situations that you believe are likely to come up from this chapter.

Special Weight Loss Situations for Women

"God places the heaviest burden on those who can carry its weight." - Reggie White

How To Boost Your Metabolism Naturally

There are a lot of people who would give a lot to increase their metabolism. Having a high level of metabolism enables one to maintain burn fat and lose weight fast with the least amount of activity. Metabolism is the rate by which the body produces and consumes energy and calories to support life.

There are several factors that affect the metabolism of a person, such as the amount of muscle tissue, the frequency of the meals you consume, genetics, stress levels, personal diet and activity levels. Metabolism slows down due to the following: loss of muscle because of not enough physical activity, the tendency of the body to cannibalize its own tissue because there is not enough food energy to sustain it, and the decrease of physical activity that often comes with older age, arthritis, and the spiral into a sedentary lifestyle.

Here are several tips to activate your metabolism:

1. **Build up on lean, mean body mass**. It is only natural that metabolism decreases along with age, but it is possible to counter the effects. The amount of muscle a person has is a very strong determinant in the ability to burn calories and shed fat.

So it goes without saying that exercise is essential. Build strength and resistance by working out at least twice a week, preferably with weights. Do easy exercises in between workouts.

Simple tasks such as walking the dog and using the stairs in place of the elevator can already take off calories. The key is to match the amount of eating to the amount of activity you have. Here are some guidelines in getting the right exercise:

For strength training:

-Increase the number of repetitions of a particular exercise.

-Add the level of resistance

-Utilize advance exercise techniques if possible

For cardiovascular training

-Insert intervals between exercises

-Perform cross-training and combine the exercises

-Add up on resistance and speed

2. **Eat breakfast**. A lot of people ignore the fact that breakfast is the most important meal of the day. Surprisingly, people who eat breakfast are thinner than the ones who do not. Metabolism can slow down considerably if breakfast is taken during mid-morning, or if one waits until the afternoon to eat. So, skipping breakfast defeats your overall goal.

3. **Avoid sugar**. Sugar enables the body to store fat. Experts recommend that you consume food that helps sustain an even level of blood-sugar. Additionally, progressive exercise 2-3 times a week should be in order to stabilize blood sugar.

4. **Eat spicy foods**. Hot cuisine with peppers can increase metabolism.

5. **Sleep more**. According to research, it is more likely for women who do not get enough sleep to gain weight. Also, muscles are regenerated during the last couple of hours of sleep at night.

6. **Increase water intake**. Water flushes out toxins that are produced whenever the body burns fat. The majority of bodily functions involve water. Lack of water causes the body system's operations to decrease their speed and produces unneeded stress as a result.

7. **Eat smaller meals**. It is advisable to consume 4 to 6 small meals that are timed 2 to 3 hours apart.

8. **Never skip meals**. People tend to skip meals in order to lose weight, which is a big mistake since it slows down metabolism.

9. **Plan meals in detail**. Always prepare the right amount of food to be consumed at the designated intervals. Do not commit the mistake of eating meals in sporadic patterns.

9. **Ditch the stress!** Stress, be it physical or emotional, triggers the release of a steroid hormone called cortisol, which decreases metabolism (and contributes to worsening diabetes, if you have a blood sugar problem). Also, people tend to eat excessively when stressed.

Take a look at the tools we suggest elsewhere in this book – hypnosis, meditation, yoga, and acupuncture. These drug-free approaches can help support you in many ways, including reducing how intensively you react when stressors show up in your life.

10. **Drink green tea several times per day.** It can be used as a substitute for coffee. Tea has the ability to stimulate metabolism (and provides health-promoting antioxidants too). Unlike coffee, tea has less caffeine to cause jittery side effects when too much is consumed. Of course you can also use decaf green tea to avoid caffeine if you are extremely sensitive to its effects.

11. **Include more energy foods and super foods in your diet**, such as fruits and vegetables, beans and whole grains.

Achieving the desired body weight is never impossible if you have the determination and patience needed to stabilize your metabolism level. Metabolism plays an important role in weight loss. Realize that eating right and working out are not just passing fancies, but a healthier way of life to give you more energy, cope easily with the ups and downs of everyday life, and to feel better overall.

Losing Weight After Pregnancy

Let's get honest with weight gain in pregnancy. You are supposed to to gain weight. You are nurturing a baby inside you who needs to develop and grow for 9 months. You need to eat for two (more if you have twins or triplets, of course).

But, once you have delivered the baby, you probably want to get your weight back to normal. On average, women lose about 10 pounds during childbirth itself.

Then over the early time period after delivering your baby, you will find that more weight will come off because of getting rid of additional fluids.

Here are some tips for losing weight after pregnancy:

1. **Focus on what you changed in your eating habits to support the pregnancy**. You are again just eating for one. Adjust your eating habits as we discussed elsewhere to get on track.

Reduce your portions.

And - No more excuses that pregnancy has caused some cravings against which you are "helpless." You are in charge – take charge.

2. **Add some light physical activity to your regular weekly schedule**. As we discussed for exercise in general, walking is a great way to ease into this part of your lifestyle.

3. **Re-tone your abdominal muscles**. Since your abdominal muscles took a big stretch "hit"for months, talk

with a personal trainer about the best way to restore tone in your abdominal muscles.

Avoiding Weight Gain in Menopause

Talking to most women over 50, you will quickly discover that menopause and weight gain are linked in their experience. It is very common to put on weight at this time of life. While some of the pounds may be due to lifestyle changes, lifestyle alone does not explain why suddenly we develop a tendency to put on weight at different parts of the body, especially the abdomen, whereas any weight gained when we were younger tends to be centered on the hips.

The truth is that hormonal changes do have a part to play in this, although the process is not completely understood. At menopause a woman stops ovulating, her monthly menstruation periods end, and her body produces much lower levels of the female hormone estrogen which is responsible for the ovulation process.

Low estrogen has been shown to cause weight gain in animals and it almost certainly is the reason why our bodies change shape during and after menopause. Another hormone, DHEA, also drops with age and may contribute to some of the issues with changes in your body (and mood).

While women of childbearing age store fat in the lower body, after the menopause they store it on the abdomen instead, like men. This leads to a greater risk of heart disease.

At the same time, both men and women tend to find muscle turning to fat as they grow older, and the metabolism slows down. This means that if you do not adjust your eating habits you will probably find that your weight increases. A person at age 60 just does not need as many calories as a person at age 40.

Hormone therapy with estrogen is sometimes prescribed to control menopausal symptoms. Estrogen has its own significant risks. Some women go to naturopaths for bioidentical hormones instead of the horse urine-derived version of estrogen that some of the conventional drugs contain.

Many women will be surprised to hear that studies have shown that hormone therapy does not cause weight gain.

Some women experience bloating and water retention in the early stages of hormone therapy but this is usually temporary and they have not gained any fat.

Hormone therapy alters your risk of heart disease by preventing the changes in storage of body fat around the abdomen and lowering cholesterol. However, hormone therapy has been linked to an increased risk of breast cancer in some studies. It is a difficult decision, and finding other ways to deal with weight gain and menopausal symptoms without using hormones may be preferable.

As always, talk with your own doctor about what is best in your personal situation.

If you find that you are gaining weight around the menopause, there are several things you can do.

- Eat a healthy, low fat diet with plenty of fiber, avoiding sugar.

- Take regular exercise. As people get older their physical activity levels naturally drop. Work often becomes less physically demanding, and there are no kids to run around after. We take less active holidays and do things more slowly. Getting 30 minutes of moderate physical activity every day will help to balance out the effect of these changes.

- Maintain your muscle strength and mass. Use weights for arm muscles and walking or cycling for legs.

- Accept the changes to the shape of your body. If you are not overweight, but simply have a thicker waist and slimmer legs, that is fine.

Consult with your doctor before starting any diet or exercise program. This is especially important if you have any medical conditions or your fitness levels are low. Your doctor can also help with symptoms of the menopause and weight gain.

Visit a naturopathic doctor for even more tips.

Consider finding a local naturopath who will have several natural remedy solutions to try instead of synthetic drugs or hormones.

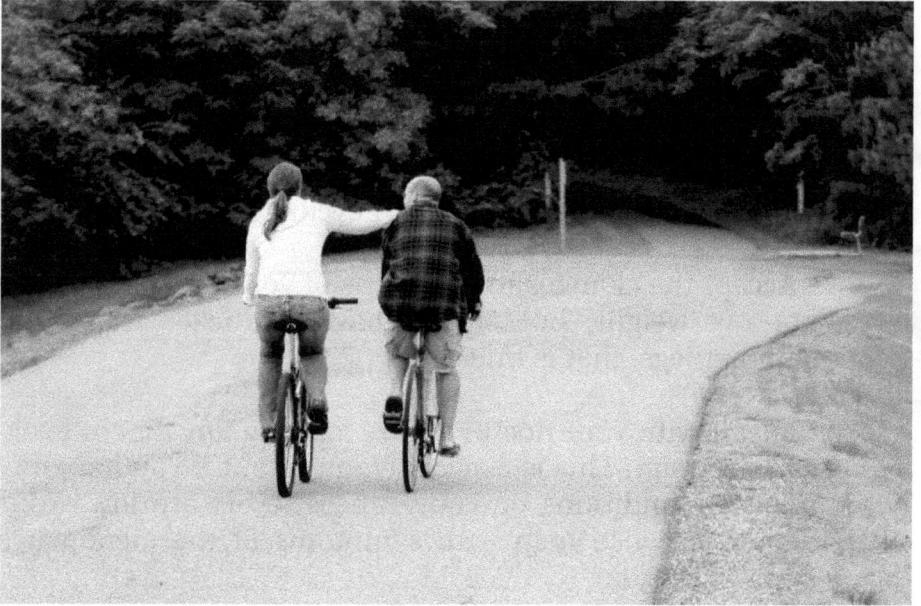

Positive Affirmations for Women

"Optimism is the foundation of courage." -- Nicholas Murray Butler

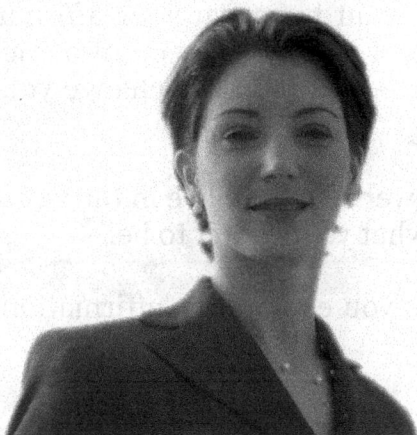

Positive affirmations are a simple but powerful way to support your decision to start a healthy diet -- and maintain the determination to stick to your diet.

An affirmation is a statement or even a solemn declaration that something is true in the present moment, the "now." Many experts in the self-growth arena encourage you to add positive affirmations to your arsenal of tools. Affirmations can put you into the right mindset for the changes you want to make in your life.

By affirming something in your mind and your emotions, you reinforce its reality for you. It is a kind of self-hypnosis or visualization. Even if you are somewhat cyni-cal about this process as "just wishful thinking," there is plenty of evidence that our behavior and even our biology fall in line with our perceptions, expectations, and beliefs.

If you perceive something to be true, you will experience your world in accord with your perceptions, expectations, and beliefs. All of that influences your life in thousands of ways of which you are aware and unaware. So, consider the expression "fake it until you make it." Be a great ac-tress in your own life and take on the part of the winner (no matter what you may have believed about yourself in the past). Affirm your intention to succeed now.

Declare yourself to be a healthy eater, a successful dieter, a strong person with self-confidence. Then behave "as if" it were already true. You'll want to repeat your affirma-tions daily and give it at least 21 days to seep into your consciousness and behavior -- and help you change your lifestyle habits.

Behaving "as if" is a very powerful way to live in the world and to shape your life into what you want it to be.

Keep these ideas in mind as you explore the affirmations below:

I make good food choices that keep me healthy.

Eating right is important. These choices are easy and worth the cost, because my health is valuable to me. I choose to eat nutritiously and make good food choices. *I like healthy food,* and purchasing and preparing it is a joy to me.

Each and every day, I eat nutritious foods, occasionally allowing myself an unhealthy treat. Everything in moderation is a good motto for me when it comes to eating healthy.

Foods that are healthy also taste good. Since there are so many choices, there is always something good to eat. I enjoy trying a wide variety of foods. The beauty is that there are still healthy fruits, vegetables, and other dishes that I haven't even tasted yet. I enjoy trying new recipes that fuel my body for success.

Healthy food is one of the best things I can give myself. It keeps me at an optimum weight and makes me feel good.

Good health is priceless and also one of the best gifts I could ever give my family. So it is important for me to prepare healthy meals for my family and teach them to make good food choices as well.

Each week, I take time to plan healthy meals; therefore I make good choices at the grocery store. I cook meals in advance and freeze them to ensure I can have healthy meals even if my schedule is hectic. For snacks, I always have plenty of healthy choices readily available to just grab and eat.

Today, I focus on eating well for optimal health.

Self-Reflection Questions:

1. What can I do today to ensure I eat well to stay healthy?
2. How can I encourage my family to follow healthy eating habits?

3. What is the best way for me to continue to improve my eating habits?

I actively seek out relaxation in my life.

I create an atmosphere of relaxation within my life.

Instead of waiting for a time to sit back and relax, I proactively make this time for myself. I am aware of my schedule and I make time for special activities that I find relaxing. By scheduling time to do the things that recharge my spirit, I become a more centered person.

I pay attention to how busy I allow myself to get and I ensure time is allotted to do the things I enjoy doing. *I allow myself to rearrange my schedule to make me a high priority*. Whether it is taking an hour in the evening to soak in a warm tub of bubbles with a glass of wine and a good book, or taking a peaceful stroll through the park, I make time for myself.

My time and my schedule are important, however, my serenity and relaxation is equally important to me. This is why I purposefully make time to step away from my busy life and simply breathe in calmness.

Today I choose to create the time I need to seek relaxation. I may simply need a half hour to feel recharged and *today I will schedule this time for myself*.

Self-Reflection Questions:

1. When managing my time have I allotted relaxation time?
2. What activities do I find relaxing?

124

3. How will I devote 20 minutes a day to relaxing?

My body deserves to be nourished and satisfied with healthy fuels.

I take care of my body because it is the only one I have. As a gift from my Creator, my body deserves to be treated with dignity and respect.

I am the only person accountable for what goes into my body. I take that responsibility very seriously because I want to keep it nourished and satisfied in order to be able to enjoy all other areas of life.

I eat balanced meals every day that supply my body all the nutrients it needs to function well. I follow the guidelines of what a person my age should eat. I actively research the latest information from health professionals on foods.

I choose foods that are free from pesticides and preservatives in order to keep my body clean. Before I eat, I always wash my fruits and vegetables carefully.

Daily, I reap the rewards of a healthy lifestyle through renewed strength and energy. **_When I practice healthy habits, I feel alive, alert, and happy._**

Although I enjoy food, I eat only as a necessity of living. I stay away from unhealthy social eating. My mind is strong enough for me to make dietary changes to improve my overall well-being.

When I fill up with healthy fuel, my engine runs smooth-ly. *I enjoy the expedition of life much more when my vehicle is in good repair.*

Today, I choose fuels that are healthy and I keep my body running smoothly because I am worth it.

Self-Reflection Questions:

1. What do I feed my body?
2. What are the rewards of living a healthy lifestyle?
3. Am I making wise food choices so I can enjoy a heal-thier life?

Final Words of Encouragement

"Never, never, never give up."

\-   Winston Churchill

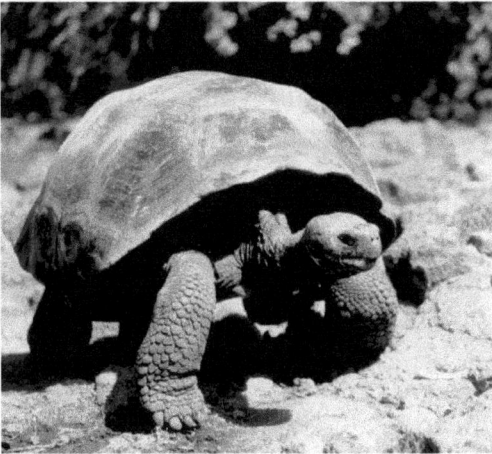

A diet is only as good or effective for you if it brings you to a better outcome than you would have without it.

You can measure the outcome in various ways – amount of weight lost, level of energy and vigor, sense of self confi-dence, ease around food, comfort wearing your clothes...whatever matters most to you.

If you've been on any diets or weight loss programs in the past then consider the results that you got from them because that is what you can expect if you go on the same diet again.

You need to look not only at the diet itself, the time that you were on it and whether you lost weight or not, but also the period after you stopped dieting. Consider how fast you put the weight back on. Very often, that weight gain after dieting was a result of the diet itself.

If you are considering another attempt at that diet where you lost a lot of weight quite rapidly, it will be worthwhile to look a little further and see what the final outcome was over the medium to long term. What happened might paint a different picture of the program and change your opinion on the effectiveness of the diet.

It might be time for you to consider an alternative way of losing weight or, to be more precise, losing fat. Losing fat is the most important thing that you should be looking at.

Consider using a weight-loss program that reduces the fat gradually and is easy to maintain while you go about your normal day-to-day life.

You might think that it will take longer to lose the weight, but what you really should be focusing on is getting to an optimum body shape and staying there for the rest of your life. Then you can be done with the yo-yo dieting ups and downs way of life.

It is not much use for you to lose weight for a few months and put it back on for the next few months -- and then repeat the cycle over and over again.

This is all that you can expect to get if that's all that you got in the past. In fact, it only becomes more difficult to lose weight and easier to put it back on. Keep that thought in your mind before you embark on another "quick" weight-loss program.

Whether this is the first time you've ever tried a diet or the 100th time, this can be your last time. When you plan ahead and set realistic goals, you'll find that sticking to your diet and maintaining a healthy lifestyle change will be possible. It also gets easier the longer you stick with it.

It starts by selecting a way of eating that will work to fit your lifestyle. What works for one person may not be appropriate for another. Don't compare yourself to anyone else – you only need to focus on your needs and your successes.

Instead of yo-yoing up and down, it's time to stick to a program that will give you what you really want.

The tortoise had it right – slow and steady wins the race. If you're in this for the long haul, you'll achieve the goals you have set for yourself. Go for it...

Your Action Steps:

1. Get started.

2. Keep going.

3. Never never never give up.

Additional Resources:

1. Get More Tools for Successful Weight Loss at:
   a. www.MasterYourMindMasterYourBody.com
   b. www.HowToStickToADiet.org

2. Learn the basics at the U.S. Government Information Site on Nutrition:
   a. www.Nutrition.gov

3. Search for a local acupuncturist at:
   a. www.AcuFinder.com

4. Find a local hypnotherapist at:
   a. www.NGH.net/referrals/request-form/

   or

   b. www.AAPH.org/directory_search

5. Check out the Personal Trainer in Your Pocket at:

   www.HowToStickToADiet.org/personal-trainer

6. Get self-hypnosis downloads to support your healthy diet and weight loss plan at:

   www.HowToStickToADiet.org/hypnosis-downloads

7. Add a good multivitamin for women to your daily diet plan at:

   www.HowToStickToADiet.org/multivitamins-for-women